SOMATIC YOGA
FOR WEIGHT LOSS

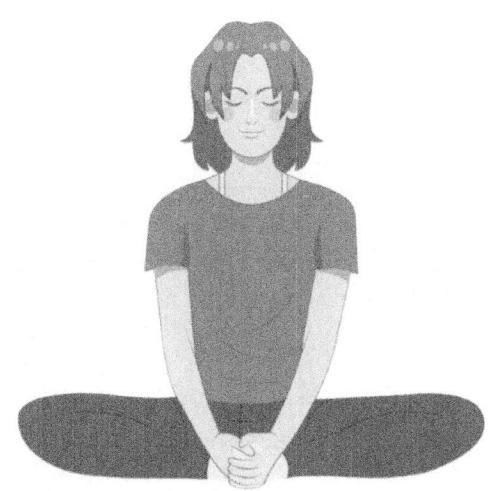

EMERSON BLAKE

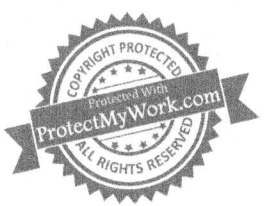

© Copyright 2023 by EMERSON BLAKE- All rights reserved.

This document is geared towards providing exact and reliable information in regard to the topic and issue covered. The publication is sold with the idea that the publisher is not required to render accounting, officially permitted, or otherwise, qualified services. If advice is necessary, legal or professional, a practiced individual in the profession should be ordered.

From a Declaration of Principles which was accepted and approved equally by a Committee of the American Bar Association and a Committee of Publishers and Associations. In no way is it legal to reproduce, duplicate, or transmit any part of this document in either electronic means or in printed format. Recording of this publication is strictly prohibited, and any storage of this document is not allowed unless with written permission from the publisher. All rights reserved.

The information provided herein is stated to be truthful and consistent, in that any liability, in terms of inattention or otherwise, by any usage or abuse of any policies, processes, or directions contained within is the solitary and utter responsibility of the recipient reader. Under no circumstances will any legal responsibility or blame be held against the publisher for any reparation, damages, or monetary loss due to the information herein, either directly or indirectly.

Respective authors own all copyrights not held by the publisher. The information herein is offered for informational purposes solely and is universal as such. The presentation of the information is without a contract or any type of guaranteed assurance. The trademarks that are used are without any consent, and the publication of the trademark is without permission or backing by the trademark owner. All trademarks and brands within this book are for clarifying purposes only and are owned by the owners themselves, not affiliated with this document.

Contents

Introduction	1
1. What is Somatic Yoga?	3
2. Why Somatic Yoga?	11
3. How to Get The Best Out of Somatic Yoga	17
4. Is 10 Minutes Enough?	28
5. Somatic Yoga 50 Illustrated Poses	34
6. 28 Days to Weight Loss and A Stress-Free Life	89
7. Tracking Your Somatic Journey	96
Conclusion	102
Exercise Index	104

Introduction

Call me what I am, which is joyful, full of life...And love...And energy and spirit. Call me what I am, and I'll tell you that I am whole.

Whole; is a word that I like, simply because it has many different meanings. Something could be whole in the sense that it's been untouched; still intact. Whole in the sense that it is organic and deeply nourishing—preservative-free, and whole in the sense that you are connected to your whole self. You are one with your body, and your body is one with you, but really, how many of us can go and stand in front of a mirror, look at ourselves, and claim ourselves as whole?

Nowadays we are constantly bombarded with a whole ton of societal pressures, from unrealistic beauty standards, and the never-ending hustle and wanting to #girlboss your way through life, all of that makes it so easy to lose touch with ourselves—our true, authentic selves. We become fragmented, disconnected from the very essence that makes us who we are. We compartmentalize our lives, segregating our professional selves from ourselves, and our physical selves from our emotional selves, and in the process, we lose sight of the interconnectedness that defines true wholeness.

What if I told you though that reclaiming that sense of wholeness is not only possible but also essential for your overall well-being? What if I said that by embracing a holistic approach, one that integrates your mind, body, and spirit, you could rediscover the joy, love, and energy that lives inside of you?

Just imagine waking up each morning feeling truly alive, your body alight with vitality, your mind clear and focused, and your spirit uplifted. Think about how liberating it would feel to move through your day with a sense of ease and grace, no longer weighed down by the burdens of stress, anxiety, or self-doubt. Picture yourself standing tall, radiating confidence and self-acceptance, because you've decided to claim the truth that you are whole, and there's nothing that can diminish that or take that away from you.

This is the very thing that somatic yoga can do for you. It's a path that recognizes that transformation is a process that starts from within and that by cultivating a deep connection with your body and honoring the wisdom that it carries, you can tap into a wellspring of lasting health, vitality, and inner peace.

Over the next couple of chapters, you're going to learn how to listen to the subtle whispers of your body, and to attune yourself to its unique rhythms and needs. You'll discover that your body is not an enemy to be conquered or a vessel to be shaped according to someone else's ideals, but rather a sacred temple, a vessel of pure strength and beauty, deserving of reverence and care.

These exercises are going to help you release layers of tension, both physical and emotional, that have accumulated over years of pushing, striving, and ignoring your body's signals. With each exhale, you'll let go of the beliefs, patterns, and conditioning that have kept you trapped in cycles of self-criticism and dissatisfaction. You are going to learn what it means to hold space for all of who you are, to celebrate your curves and your strength, and to honor the incredible journey your body has been on and the stories it has to tell. You're going to learn to hold space for the truth that genuine beauty lies in the radiant glow that comes from living in alignment with your authentic self, one breath, one movement, one moment of self-acceptance at a time because when we are whole, we are unstoppable, capable of anything our hearts desire.

Chapter One

What is Somatic Yoga?

Now when I tell you that I have just about tried every kind of weight loss, believe me. From keto to low carb, the juice cleanses, I have even gone so far as to starve myself half to death and only eat a piece of string cheese when it feels like I'm going to pass out kind of diet.

I've been there, done that, and bought the overpriced t-shirt, and let me tell you, none of those fads brought me any lasting joy or peace with my body. In fact, they only deepened the rift between my physical self and my mental well-being, leaving me trapped in a cycle of deprivation, guilt, and self-loathing. Can you remember a time when you stood in front of the mirror, pinching at your flesh, scrutinizing every supposed flaw and imperfection? When the number on the scale dictated your entire mood for the day, a lower number bringing fleeting elation, but a higher one plunging you into depths of despair?

I know I can. Those memories are etched into my mind, reminders of the dark days when I viewed my body as an enemy to be conquered, a problem to be solved, rather than the sacred vessel that carries me through this life. Then, after another failed attempt, something shifted, a small voice within me began to whisper, "Enough. There has to be a better way." And that's when I started thinking about the idea that weight loss doesn't have to be a battle, but can instead be a loving, nurturing journey of self-discovery and self-acceptance. Imagine that—treating your body with kindness, compassion, and respect, rather than punishing it with deprivation and self-hatred. Embracing the notion that true health and vitality come not from adhering to rigid rules or unrealistic standards, but from tuning into the wisdom of your own being, listening to its needs, and honoring its unique rhythms.

It was a paradigm shift that shook me to my core, challenging everything I thought I knew about weight loss and body image. I realized that I didn't have to wage war against my own flesh to achieve my desired physique. Instead, I could approach the process with curiosity, gentleness, and a deep reverence for the incredible vessel that carries me through this life. Every pound shed became not a victory over my body, but a loving act of self-care, a celebration of the strength and resilience that lay within me all along.

And you know what? The weight began to melt away, not because I was depriving myself or punishing my body, but because I was finally in alignment with its true needs, nourishing it from the inside out with love, respect, and a newfound appreciation for all that it carries. Weight loss doesn't have to be a battle; it can be a labor of love, something that leads you to a place of profound peace and acceptance within your own skin.

What is Somatic Yoga?

Somatic yoga is a holistic approach that combines the principles of traditional yoga with the insights of somatics, a field that explores the mind-body connection and the lived experience of the physical self. While the main focus in traditional yoga is physical postures (asanas) and breath work (pranayama), somatic yoga looks more deeply into body awareness, movement patterns, and the interplay between our mental and physical states.

Its roots date back to the work of pioneers like Moshe Feldenkrais, Ida Rolf, and Thomas Hanna, who developed modalities such as the Feldenkrais Method, Rolfing, and Somatics, respectively. These approaches emphasized the importance of being highly aware of how we move, hold tension, and unconsciously develop habitual patterns that can cause us discomfort, pain, and imbalances within the body.

One of the main differences between somatic yoga and traditional yoga lies in the emphasis placed on proprioception, or the body's ability to sense its own movement and position in space. In somatic yoga, you're encouraged to move with mindful awareness and to pay close attention to the sensations that arise within the body as they transition from one posture to the next. This is what gives you more insight into your own unique movement patterns, areas of tension or restriction, and the interconnectedness of the physical, mental, and emotional realms.

The approach to the physical postures as well is also a factor. While traditional yoga often emphasizes achieving specific alignment and form in each asana, somatic yoga recognizes and appreciates the fact that everybody is unique, with its own limitations, strengths, and optimal ranges of motion. Instead of striving for a predetermined idealized shape, we are encouraged to look within, honor the body's innate knowledge, and find the tools and strategies that are most appropriate to us. This focus on inner exploration and self-awareness is a hallmark of somatic yoga because it empowers us to cultivate a deep sense of connection and respect for our bodies. The subtle keys and sensations teach us to respect our bodies and begin the process of releasing those long-held patterns of tension, trauma, or emotional blockages that may have manifested as physical discomfort or imbalances.

Understanding the Somatic Experience

So when our nervous systems don't feel safe enough, they can get stuck in a state of dysregulation, where we remain in a heightened state of arousal or freeze response, even after the perceived threat has passed.

Somatic experiencing is a body-oriented approach to healing trauma and resolving stuck physiological states. recognizes that trauma is not just a psychological or emotional experience, but a physiological one that also influences the autonomic nervous system and the body's instinctive responses to perceived threats; it's about understanding that the body has an innate ability to regulate and discharge the high levels of energy and activation associated with traumatic events. However, when this natural process is disrupted or incomplete, the residual energy can become trapped, leading to a wide range of physical and psychological symptoms, such as anxiety, depression, chronic pain, and dissociation.

The gentle, guided exploration of bodily sensations and subtle movements in somatic experiencing renegotiate the stuck survival responses and restore a sense of safety and equilibrium within the nervous system. This process involves carefully titrating the level of arousal, allowing the individual to gradually approach and release the stored trauma in a controlled and manageable way.

The Principles of Somatic Yoga

Somatic yoga is very practical, so it can in some way always be applied. This is the reason why it's been practiced for thousands of years and is still very much valid, even today. Here are the principles that it can be broken down into:

Body Awareness and Interoception

You cannot heal what you are not aware of, that's something that my gran always said. If you have a pain somewhere in your body, you have to investigate where that comes from and what the potential causes could be. So awareness and interoception, in this case, mean that you cultivate a heightened sense of attunement and sensitivity to the subtle cues and sensations arising within your physical form.

It's about developing a deep, intimate relationship with your body, listening to its whispers, and honoring the wisdom it holds. Too often, we move through life disconnected from our experiences, ignoring the signals our bodies send us until they manifest as chronic pain, illness, or dysfunction. Somatic yoga invites us to break this cycle by fostering a state of present, embodied awareness.

Mindful movement explorations, breath work, and guided sensory attunement practices turn our attention inward, making us attuned to the nuances of our physical sensations. We notice the areas of tension, the patterns of holding, the places where energy feels stuck or restricted, and the subtle shifts that occur as we move and breathe. Being able to interpret the messages our bodies are sending us, gives us invaluable insight into our unique needs, limitations, and imbalances. We can then respond with compassion and wisdom, adjusting our movements, postures, and practices to better support our journeys toward greater balance and well-being.

Honoring Individual Variation

You are not me, and I am not you. Our limits are simply not the same. This simple truth lies at the very heart of this principle. We each come to the practice with our unique physical structures, histories, and inherent capabilities. Using a one-size-fits-all approach or striving for a predetermined ideal form would be to deny the exquisite diversity of the human experience.

Somatic yoga recognizes and celebrates this variation, inviting us to do movements, postures, and practices from a place of deep self-knowledge and self-acceptance, instead of forcing our bodies into rigid molds, we are encouraged to listen to our individual needs, to respect our limitations while simultaneously embracing our strengths.

This principle acknowledges that what feels effortless and nourishing for one person may be a struggle or even a source of discomfort for another. It rejects the notion of a universal "correct" alignment or expression of a posture, instead encouraging us to find the variations and modifications that feel most authentic and supportive of our unique physical forms. We learn to cultivate a profound sense of self-compassion and self-trust. We shed the impulse to compare ourselves to others or to strive for an externally defined ideal, instead focusing our attention on the innate wisdom and capabilities that reside within our beings.

We also each carry our own histories, traumas, and perspectives, and these too must be honored and integrated into our practice. It empowers us to move beyond the confines of rigid expectations and to forge our unique paths toward greater well-being, vitality, and embodied presence.

Mind-Body Integration

How can you separate me from the very essence of who I am? I am one with my body and my mind, and those are one together. We are not merely physical vessels housing separate mental and emotional experiences; rather, we are complex beings created from the inseparable threads of body, mind, and spirit.

To approach the practice from a purely physical perspective would be to deny that interconnectedness that defines our human experience. Our thoughts, emotions, and mental states are constantly shaping and influencing our physical realities, just like how our bodily sensations and movements ripple outward, impacting our energetic and emotional landscapes. Somatic yoga embraces this holistic understanding, inviting us to explore the intricate dance between our physical, mental, and emotional states.

As we move and breathe with conscious presence, we may notice how emotions like anxiety or sadness manifest as physical tension or constriction. Or, we may experience how the release of long-held patterns of muscular holding can catalyze profound shifts in our emotional and mental states, unveiling layers of buried emotion or liberating us from limiting thought patterns. Mind-body integration empowers us to approach our practice as something multidimensional; it invites us to explore the landscapes that make us who we are. It attunes us to the language of our bodies, using this wisdom as a gateway to deeper self-understanding and self-acceptance.

Nervous System Regulation

When your nervous system feels safe enough to relax, safe enough to be, laugh, and love, you experience a newfound sense of presence, vitality, and connection with the world around you, however, when the balance of your nervous system is disrupted by trauma, stress, or dysregulation, it can feel like being trapped in a constant state of high alert, where even the simplest tasks or interactions are laced with tension and unease.

This principle recognizes that true healing and well-being are rooted in restoring a sense of safety and equilibrium within our autonomic nervous systems—the intricate networks that govern our unconscious processes, such as heart rate, respiration, and our innate responses to perceived threats. Somatic yoga offers a pathway to renegotiating these stuck survival responses and returning to a state of balanced regulation. We learn to attune to the subtle cues and sensations that signal dysregulation, such as shallow breathing, muscle tension, or a sense of disconnection from our bodies.

Guided by the wisdom of our own somatic experiences, we then engage in practices designed to gradually restore a sense of safety and grounding within the nervous system. This might involve breath work to activate the calming influence of the parasympathetic nervous system, or gentle rocking or swaying movements that tap into our innate, self-regulating capacities. As we move through these explorations with mindful presence, we create new neural pathways and physical patterns that communicate safety and resilience to our nervous systems. We begin to rewire our instinctive responses, trading fight-or-flight reactivity for a deeper sense of embodied presence and self-regulation.

When our nervous systems feel truly safe and balanced, we experience a palpable shift in our lived experiences. We become more present, more attuned to the richness of each moment, and more capable of experiencing the full spectrum of human emotion—from deep joy and connection to the occasional waves of sadness or discomfort.

Self-Compassion and Self-Acceptance

So many of us approach weight loss from a place of self-judgment and self-hatred that we inadvertently perpetuate cycles of shame, deprivation, and disconnection from our bodies. We berate ourselves for our flaws, punish our physical forms with harsh regimens, and measure our worth by arbitrary numbers on a scale, making us lose sight of the beauty that makes us who we are.

The principle of self-compassion and self-acceptance in somatic yoga offers a radical shift from this paradigm of self-criticism. It invites us to approach our journey towards well-being from a place of deep reverence, kindness, and unconditional love for ourselves—exactly as we are in this present moment.

At the core of this principle lies the understanding that change cannot be rooted in self-loathing or self-rejection. When we approach our practice from a space of judgment or harsh self-criticism, we create an adversarial relationship with our bodies, fostering resistance, shame, and a perpetual sense of never being "enough." But when we welcome self-compassion and self-acceptance, we create an environment conducive to growth, healing, and profound self-discovery. We learn to treat our bodies with the same tender care and respect we would extend to a beloved friend or family member, acknowledging our strengths and limitations with equal compassion.

This lens of self-love helps shed the limiting beliefs, societal conditioning, and unrealistic expectations that have long governed and held our relationships with our physical forms prisoner. We learn to celebrate the bodies that have held us, honoring the stories etched into every curve, every scar, every imperfection that bears witness to our lived experiences. It's not just about body positivity; it is a deep, unwavering commitment to valuing and cherishing ourselves in our entirety – our minds, our emotions, our spirits, and the exquisite vessels that house them all.

Presence and Embodied Awareness

Learning to love our bodies is simply about learning to honor them for what they are in the moment, this moment right now... We are too disconnected from the here and now, our minds are constantly projecting into the future or ruminating on the past. We are chasing after idealized versions of ourselves or clinging to outdated narratives that no longer serve us. Somatic yoga calls us to inhabit our bodies fully, to attune to the subtle sensations and experiences unfolding within our physical selves with each breath, each movement, each heartbeat; to let go of the need to judge, interpret, or intellectualize, and instead, we must just be here to bear witness to the ever-changing landscape of our somatic existence.

When we can do that, we become more present–a quality of being that transcends the limitations of language and conceptual thought. We become intimately attuned to the nuances of our physical sensations, the ebb and flow of our breath, and the intricate interplay between our bodies and the world around us. We unwrap layers that have long been obscured by the relentless chatter of our minds. We learn to honor and celebrate the stories etched into every curve, every scar, every imperfection that bears witness to our lived experiences. It is an invitation to move beyond the constraints of our analytical minds and to experience the world through the raw, visceral lens of our embodied existence—a perspective that awakens reverence for the miracle that is our human form.

The Role of Breathing in Somatic Yoga

If you're a runner or you have spent time in the gym, you'll know that how, when, and how you breathe is extremely important. Proper breathing is just as crucial for somatic yoga practice. Breathing techniques play several key roles:

- Breath awareness. Many somatic yoga practices begin by simply tuning into the breath and noticing your natural breathing patterns. This cultivates mind-body awareness and presence.

- Relaxation. Controlled breathing, such as extended exhales, can trigger the parasympathetic nervous system responsible for resting and digesting. This reduces stress and anxiety.

- Energy control. Specific breathing patterns like breath retention are used to build heat/energy or bring a calming influence during yoga postures.

Some common breathing techniques in somatic yoga include:

- Dirga Pranayama (Three-Part Breath) - This involves deepening the breath by consciously expanding the lower abdomen, rib cage, and upper chest on the inhale.

- Nadi Shodhana (Alternate Nostril Breathing) - Alternating nostril breathing, is said to balance the mind and purify the subtle energy channels.

- Kapalabhati (Skull Shining Breath) - A forced exhale created by contracting the lower abdomen. It builds heat, focus, and cleanses.

- Bhastrika (Bellows Breath) - A vigorous breath combining inhales and exhales through the nose. It increases metabolic fire and oxygenation.

Proper breathing integrates the mind and body in somatic yoga. Different techniques can be used to prepare for postures, enhance awareness, or provide specific energetic benefits during the practice.

Chapter Two
Why Somatic Yoga?

So whenever you are about to start something, one of the most important questions to ask yourself is why you are doing it. So all those years back when I went on all those fad diets, the "why" behind my reasoning was always so short-sighted and superficial—to simply lose weight as quickly as possible.

The first one was one of those extreme low-carb plans that was all the rage at the time. For the first few weeks, the pounds just melted off. I felt accomplished, in control, and determined to finally conquer my body issues once and for all. But it didn't take long for the intense cravings to set in—for a piece of bread, a bowl of rice, a measly little cookie. My willpower wavered as hunger pangs took over, but before I knew it, I had fallen off the wagon completely, binging on all the foods I had been depriving myself of. The weight piled back on even faster than it had come off. Worse yet, I felt like an utter failure—ashamed, disappointed in myself, and completely demoralized. Why did I do this to myself again?

The cycle repeated itself more times than I care to admit—an unsustainable diet, unrealistic restrictions, inevitable deprivation followed by binging, self-loathing, weight cycling up and down. Each time left me more frustrated, disconnected from my body, and obsessed with the number on the scale. Many years later, I finally began to understand the real, profound "why" behind my quest for better health and weight loss. It went far beyond merely changing my outer appearance, it was about learning to love and appreciate my body, not for what it can be, but for all that it already is.

A Holistic Approach to Wellness

Holistic means taking into account the complete or whole of something, rather than just treating or focusing on separate parts. Wellness goes beyond just physical health—it encompasses multiple dimensions of well-being including mental, emotional, spiritual, social, and environmental aspects. A holistic approach to wellness means addressing your whole being—mind, body, and spirit—not just zeroing in on weight loss or physical fitness alone. Somatic yoga embraces this holistic philosophy in several key ways:

First, the "somatic" part refers to the mind-body connection. Somatic practices help you become deeply aware of how your physical body and psychological/emotional state are intimately intertwined. You learn to listen to the inner cues, sensations, and intuition of your body rather than just pushing it into idealized shapes from the outside.

There are also breathing exercises, meditation, visualization, and mindfulness elements that target the mental/emotional aspects of wellness. Practices like breathwork and meditation have been shown to reduce stress, anxiety, and depression and promote resilience. The spirituality component of holistic wellness is also addressed through somatic yoga's roots in Eastern philosophy and energy principles. You become attuned to the energy systems of the body and the subtle forces of awareness and presence.

Somatic therapy works not only on the physical body but also integrates techniques for self-study, introspection, and personal growth. This sets the stage for true, lasting wellness on all levels.

Empowerment and Weight Loss Through Self-Discovery

You know that feeling—when you look in the mirror and that mean little voice starts criticizing and tearing you down? "You're so fat and disgusting. You'll never be good enough until you lose this weight." That bully lives rent-free in so many of our heads, perpetuating harmful stories about our worthiness being tied to a number on the scale. What if instead of just focusing on shedding unwanted pounds, we looked at weight loss through a bigger lens? What if we saw it as an opportunity to unearth, unravel, and ultimately shed the toxic beliefs, assumptions, and narratives that we've internalized and allowed to shape our self-perception over the years?

Here's the hard truth that many of us need to hear: diets don't just help us lose physical weight, they force us to lose parts of ourselves and not the bad parts that we want to let go of, but too often the good parts too—our ability to trust our bodies' intuition, to feel comfortable experiencing true hunger, to eat from a place of nourishment rather than deprivation.

Somatic yoga is about regaining our birthright of being an embodied, conscious, and empowered human being first helps us come back home to ourselves by inviting us to self-study, to be compassionate, and to embrace the imperfect and beautiful reality of our lived experiences.

It's saying "I don't just want to change how I look, I want to change how I see myself from the inside out." It's permitting yourself to question the stories you've inherited about not being thin enough, attractive enough, or worthy enough. It's a courageous examination of how you use food and your body image to distract from facing the harder emotional work you need to do. At the end of it all, it's all about learning how to let go—letting go of the shaming monologues, brushing aside societal ideals of beauty, disconnecting from your intuition, and living by restrictive rules. It's a repositioning, a rewiring until your body is no longer an object to criticize, deprive, and attempt to manipulate into something it's not... but a loved vessel to inhabit fully, to experience life's highest and richest moments because only when we can make peace with ourselves exactly as we are, can we finally experience true, sustainable, embodied transformation, the kind that goes far deeper than physical weight loss alone.

The Role of Self-Awareness

At its core, somatic yoga isn't just about contorting your body into pretzel shapes. It's about intimately exploring who you are from the inside out, a brave encounter with all those hidden parts of yourself that you may have spent years avoiding or numbing out from.

True self-awareness requires the courage to pause, go inward, and get radically real with yourself. It means peeling back the layers of who you think you're supposed to be, the stories you've unconsciously accepted about your worth, and awakening to your authentic self. Somatic practices build this self-awareness in a few powerful ways. First, there's the subtle body attunement that happens when you sync your conscious mind with the felt experiences and psychophysical cues within. Instead of pushing or forcing, you learn to listen to and respect your body's innate wisdom.

Then there are the mindfulness and meditation elements that train you to witness your thoughts, emotions, and self-talk with compassionate non-judgment. You become intimately acquainted with your inner critic's monologues and can choose to challenge those toxic narratives. The breath awareness that's central to somatic yoga also anchors you firmly in the present moment reality rather than letting your mind wander to the future or past. This cultivates an awakened presence and embodied self-consciousness. Then perhaps most importantly, it creates a space of unconditional self-acceptance and self-discovery without agenda. There's no traditional choreography to "get right." Instead, each practice is an unfolding exploration of your unique bodily experiences, boundaries, and bodily-felt truths.

With this level of self-study comes profound growth and empowerment. You learn to show up for yourself fully—not just the curated, socially acceptable parts, but all the messy, beautifully imperfect parts too. And in doing so, you begin living with unshakable authenticity, self-trust, and freedom.

So while weight loss may be one outcome, the larger reward of somatic yoga is the clarity, confidence, and deep self-awareness that arises from truly knowing—and being yourself.

The Principles of Self-Awareness

But how exactly do you build that level of attunement? It starts with embodying a few key principles.

The first is giving yourself full permission to feel. So often, we've learned to numb, ignore, or override the subtle signals our bodies send us. But tuning into physical sensations like tightness, tingling, or expansiveness provides rich insight. During a somatic practice, you might notice your shoulders creeping toward your ears and realize you're carrying unprocessed stress. Or perhaps your belly feels tight and constricted, mirroring how you've been anxiously bracing against uncertainty. With focused awareness, you can then consciously soften those emotional-somatic patterns.

Developing a beginner's mindset is another pillar, so basically, let go of preconceived judgments, assumptions, and identification with your personal story. For example, if you habitually critique your body with thoughts like "My arms are too flabby" or "I hate my belly rolls," you practice seeing your form through fresh, curious eyes during somatic yoga—not from a place of harsh self-criticism.

Then you tend to your inner experience versus outer performance. Rather than getting caught up in perfectly mimicking yoga postures, you learn to notice: "Where does this shape create tension or ease in my body? What am I instinctively compensating for or resisting against?" The postures become a frank dialogue between your body's unique holdings and habits.

Stress and Weight Gain

My go-to when I'm feeling stressed is a tub of Ben and Jerry's ice cream. I know I'm not alone in turning to food for comfort when life feels overwhelming. But that compulsive eating often leads to weight gain, which then causes more stress, perpetuating an unhealthy cycle.

The truth is, stress takes both a physical and mental toll that can sabotage even the best weight loss efforts. On a physical level, constant high stress triggers the release of cortisol, known as the "stress hormone." Cortisol causes the body to go into survival mode, sending signals to accumulate extra fat stores, especially around the abdomen. It also increases appetite and drives cravings for sugary, fatty foods.

Stress also dysregulates other hormones like leptin and ghrelin that control hunger and feelings of fullness. This makes you more likely to overeat past the point of satiety. Mentally and emotionally, stress manifests as anxiety, depression, and low self-esteem—states in which we're more prone to engage in mindless emotional eating as a coping mechanism.

Then there's the impact stress has on our activity levels and motivation. When we are flooded with stress hormones, we tend to conserve energy and move less than usual. Exercise starts seeming like an insurmountable burden rather than self-care. The combination of increased appetite, reduced physical activity, and hormonal imbalance creates the perfect conditions for weight gain.

This is where somatic yoga helps us break the vicious stress-weight gain cycle. Gentle yoga flows, meditation, pranayama breathwork, and conscious relaxation all help reduce stress by lowering cortisol levels and calming the nervous system. As the mind-body awareness heightens, you become more attuned to emotional hunger cues versus true physical hunger.

The self-study and self-compassion aspects of somatic yoga also encourage you to address the root stressors or emotional triggers that spur compulsive behaviors like overeating. You learn to process difficult emotions through your body in a healthy way rather than seeking solace in food. Additionally, its emphasis on tuning into sensation disrupts patterns of numbing out through excessive eating. Feeling fullness and satiety become an embodied, intrinsic practice rather than simply following external rules.

When we lower stress and develop inner attunement, we move more towards a healthy lifestyle. We step off the weight gain-diet cycle not by waging war with your body, but by befriending it from the inside-out. That's the beauty of the somatic approach to well-being.

Chapter Three

How to Get The Best Out of Somatic Yoga

I have always been the best at getting "the best out of things", so to say. Whether it was finding the most cost-effective deals, maximizing value, or squeezing every ounce of excitement from an experience—I had a knack for it. I guess it's a trait that I inherited from my dad.

Growing up, he was the ultimate opportunist and master negotiator. At restaurants, he would politely inquire about any dishes not on the menu that the chef could whip up from ingredients they had. Buying a new car? You can bet he spent months researching every possible combo to get the perfect trim and features for the lowest price.

His relentless quest for unlocking hidden potential extended to our vacations too. Dad would pore over local blogs and insider guides to sniff out all the off-the-beaten-path gems, hole-in-the-wall eateries, and secret vantage points that most tourists overlooked. Thanks to his efforts, even a weekend road trip morphed into an epic adventure.

I admired the way he approached life with such intentionality and resourcefulness. Nothing was ever taken at face value—he was always peeling back layers, making unexpected connections, and figuring out how to unearth opportunities that others missed. It rubbed off on me.

In college, I became that friend who knew all the underrated takeout spots and best happy hour deals. At work, I'm the one finding creative life hacks to level up processes. My family jokes that I never do anything at "half-capacity." I'm stubbornly determined to maximize every situation.

While it can sometimes verge on obsessiveness, this drive to constantly explore, optimize, and experience things to the fullest has enriched my life immeasurably. It's kept me curious, and resourceful, and opened my eyes to possibilities I may have overlooked. And it's this same energy I brought to somatic yoga and uncovering its deepest potential.

Setting Intentions and Goals

You always gotta have a "why" because your why is what is going to keep you going when the motivation is completely non-existent. Your why is what's going to propel you forward and remind you of your deeper purpose when challenges arise.

This is especially true for something like somatic yoga, which requires an investment of time, energy, and commitment. If your only goal is to "lose weight" that motivation can quickly fizzle out when the number on the scale isn't budging, but if your intention goes beyond the surface level, it becomes an anchor to return to.

Maybe your "why" is to heal your relationship with your body after years of harsh criticism. Or to find freedom from food and body obsession. Perhaps it's to build unshakeable self-confidence from the inside out. When you tap into these bigger purposeful drivers, the practice itself becomes the reward, not just weight loss.

That's why it's so vital to get clear on your core goals and driving intentions before embarking on this somatic yoga journey. Don't just fall into it aimlessly. Pause and reflect: What are you hoping to manifest in your life? What does living in alignment with your most empowered and authentic self look and feel like?

From there, you can set "SMART" goals: Specific, Measurable, Attainable, Relevant, Time-bound...and have them be Yours. Vague resolutions like "get healthier" won't motivate you nearly as much as "I will practice somatic yoga 3 times per week for 60 days to increase my body awareness and self-compassion."

With your goal clearly defined, you can then explore the core desires and emotional drivers that led you to that intention. Perhaps regaining body wisdom heals repeated cycles of disordered eating. Self-acceptance frees you from the limiting narratives holding you back.

When you are deliberate, intentional, and granular about your whys and what you're working towards, your practice no longer becomes just a random routine - it's a lifeline anchored to your deepest values. You'll find yourself coming to your mat not just begrudgingly but with purposeful presence and a sense of it being a ritual of realignment. Your intentions keep you on track and make the journey not only productive but deeply resonant.

Tips on Setting Your Intentions

Step 1: Get quiet and go inward

This is your time to tune into the subtle feelings, desires, and intuitive nudges that often get drowned out by external noise.

Step 2: Reflect on your "whys"

With a soft gaze inward, think deeply about why you feel called to this somatic yoga journey right now. What areas of your life or sense of self feel out of alignment or unfulfilled? Are you seeking healing from negative body image, freedom from food fixation, more self-love, and confidence? Get granular about your core motivators.

Step 3: Explore your vision

Now expand that perspective into a vivid mental picture of what your life looks like when you achieve those aims. Imagine your relationship to your body, the way you move through the world, your emotional landscape. What would it feel like to exist in that realized state of being? Let the details energize your consciousness.

Step 4: Clarify your intentions

From that vision, the intentions start taking shape. Maybe your intention is "I am embodying unshakeable confidence and self-assurance." Or "I receive and trust my body's innate wisdom." Let these phrases crystalize as potent reminders of your purpose. Write them down to provide anchors.

Step 5: Set specific, resonant goals

With your driving intentions laid out, you can now set goals that align with and support those aims. Be as specific as possible with process-based outcomes you can track. For example: "I will commit to a daily 20-minute somatic yoga and breathwork practice to cultivate resilient self-trust."

Step 6: Identify obstacles

Bring awareness to any potential obstacles, resistance patterns, or past false starts that could arise and derail your goals. Lack of time management? Activated emotional triggers? Name them so you can proactively develop strategies to work through them.

Step 7: Create accountability

How are you going to ensure that you stay the course? This could involve setting calendar reminders, finding a practice partner, or scheduling check-ins to review your progress. Added accountability increases follow-through.

Step 8: Begin your practice

With your powerful intentions now inscribed, approach each somatic yoga session as a ritual to lean into those aims more deeply. Use the opening and closing moments to restate your core drivers. This attunement turns routine into living resonance.

The key is making this an embodied, deeply personal process of self-inquiry and soul-nurturing rather than jotting down a superficial weight-loss goal. Doing this work allows your somatic practice to unfold as a sacred offering in service of your highest self.

Creating a Supportive Environment

Positive environments have a direct impact on our ability to fully immerse ourselves in the present moment and reap the maximum benefits. Just like a child who grows up in a nurturing home filled with love and safety develops into a confident, self-assured adult with healthy boundaries, surrounding ourselves with an atmosphere that fosters positivity, comfort, and acceptance lays the foundation for personal growth and transformation.

When we feel seen, heard, and respected—whether by a loving partner or within the sacred space we've crafted for our practice—we find it easier to let our guards down, embracing our authentic selves without judgment or inhibition. This openness allows us to dive deeper into the somatic experience, tapping into the mind-body connection with greater clarity and intention.

Creating a supportive environment for your somatic yoga practice is like laying fertile soil for a garden to thrive. With the proper elements in place, you create the ideal conditions for self-exploration, healing, and personal growth to take root and blossom.

Preparing for Your Practice

Your ideal environment is about nurturing multiple aspects of your physical and mental space. Here are some key elements to focus on, along with detailed examples:

Physical Space:

- Your space should be a haven: calming, comfortable, and free from distractions. This could be a quiet corner of your home, a serene room, or even an outdoor space surrounded by nature.

- Ensure proper lighting, either through natural light or soft, warm lamps that create a soothing ambiance.

- Consider the temperature and ventilation to avoid feeling too hot or too cold during your practice.

- Use props like yoga mats, blankets, pillows, and blocks to support your body and enhance your comfort.

- Incorporate elements of nature, such as plants, crystals, or a small water feature, to bring a sense of tranquility and connection to the natural world.

Sensory Experience:

- Create a calming soundscape by playing gentle instrumental music, or nature sounds, or utilizing a white noise machine to block out external noises.

- Incorporate aromatherapy by burning natural candles or using essential oil diffusers with scents that promote relaxation, such as lavender, chamomile, or sandalwood.

- Engage your sense of sight by placing visually pleasing items like artwork, inspirational quotes, or images of nature around your practice space.

Personal Rituals:

- Establish a consistent practice routine, whether it's a specific time of day or a regular day of the week, to reinforce the habit and create a sense of familiarity.

- Develop a pre-practice routine that helps you transition into a mindful state, such as taking a few deep breaths, reciting a mantra, or engaging in a brief meditation.

- After your practice, allow yourself time to slowly integrate back into your daily life, perhaps by journaling, drinking a warm beverage, or simply sitting in stillness for a few moments.

Emotional Support:

- Surround yourself with reminders of your intentions, values, and aspirations through affirmations, vision boards, or meaningful objects.

- Create a sacred space by including items that hold personal significance, such as photographs, mementos, or symbols of your spiritual beliefs.

- Consider involving loved ones or a supportive community in your practice by sharing your journey, seeking encouragement, or practicing together when possible.

Mental Preparation:

- Before beginning your practice, take a few moments to mentally clear any distractions or worries that may be lingering in your mind.

- Use visualization techniques to imagine yourself in a peaceful and supportive environment, free from judgment or external pressures.

- Set a specific intention for your practice, whether it's cultivating self-acceptance, releasing tension, or simply being present in the moment.

Progressing Safely and Gradually

Somatic yoga, as simple and gentle as it may appear, requires care and safety considerations to truly harness its transformative power. While the practice encourages deep exploration of the mind-body connection through mindful movements and breathwork, you have to take into consideration your limitations. Progressing gradually not only minimizes the risk of physical injuries but also fosters a solid foundation of body awareness, proprioception, and mind-body integration – the very cornerstones upon which the profound benefits of somatic yoga are built. When you let yourself first build up momentum and then take it up from there, you create the most ideal environments for you to thrive. Here are a few more reasons why.

Injury Prevention:

Gentle movements, breath work, and body awareness exercises are all things we explore but even seemingly simple practices can pose risks if not approached with care and proper alignment. Progressing gradually allows your body to adapt to new movements, build strength and flexibility at a sustainable pace, and minimize the risk of strains, sprains, or other injuries.

Respecting Individual Limitations:

We are all built differently and each has unique physical abilities, limitations, and experiences. Some may have pre-existing conditions, injuries, or mobility issues that require extra caution and modifications. Taking a step-by-step approach allows you to tune into your body's unique needs, respect its boundaries, and avoid pushing beyond your current capabilities, which could lead to discomfort or potential harm.

Building a Solid Foundation:

Somatic yoga is not just about physical postures; it emphasizes developing a deep understanding of your body's patterns, habits, and areas of tension or imbalance. A slow and steady approach allows you to cultivate body awareness, proprioception (the sense of your body's position and movement), and mind-body integration. This solid foundation is essential for advancing safely and effectively in your practice.

Cultivating Mindfulness and Presence:

A key aspect of somatic yoga is being present at the moment and deeply attuned to the sensations and experiences within your body. Rushing through practices or advancing too quickly can lead to disconnection from this mindful state, diminishing the benefits of the practice and increasing the risk of mindless movements that may compromise safety.

Honoring the Journey:

Somatic yoga is not just about achieving specific physical goals; it's a kind of personal growth undertaking. Progressing gradually encourages patience, self-compassion, and a recognition that the process itself is incredibly valuable. With a gentle, step-by-step approach, you honor the nature of the practice and allow yourself to fully integrate its lessons.

Avoiding Injury

An unplanned or unexpected injury can derail your progress. I remember my "bad-ass" CrossFit girly stage. I'd go full steam 7 days a week—little to no rest days in between. I was riding high on the endorphin rush and the sense of accomplishment that came with pushing my body to its limits. However, my gung-ho approach eventually caught up with me. One day, during a particularly intense WOD (Workout of the Day), I felt a sharp twinge in my lower back as I was mid-rep on a heavy deadlift. Ignoring the warning signals, I powered through the workout, only to wake up the next morning barely able to move without searing pain.

That dreaded lower back injury sidelined me for weeks, forcing me to miss workouts and robbing me of the progress I had worked so hard to achieve. When I gingerly made my way through recovery, I realized the hard truth: my "no pain, no gain" mentality had been misguided. Pushing past my body's limits without proper rest and recovery had not only stalled my fitness journey but also put me at risk of more severe, long-term consequences.

It was a humbling lesson and from that point on, I vowed to prioritize gradual progression, proper form, and adequate rest, recognizing that true strength and growth come not from reckless abandon but from a mindful, holistic approach to movement and self-care.

Avoiding Injury During Cool Downs and Warm Ups

Warm-Up

- Start slowly: Begin with gentle movements and gradually increase the intensity to prepare your body for the upcoming practice. Rushing into strenuous activities can lead to strains and pulls.

- Focus on mobility: Do dynamic stretches and joint rotations to increase blood flow, lubricate your joints, and improve your range of motion. This can help prevent tightness and stiffness during your practice.

- Activate your muscles: Engage in light, controlled movements that target the major muscle groups you'll be using during your practice. This "wakes up" those muscles and prepares them for the work ahead.

- Breathe deeply: Conscious breathing not only oxygenates your muscles but also helps you connect with your body and cultivate a mindful state for your practice.

Cool-Down

- Allocate sufficient time: Don't rush through your cool-down. Allow at least 5-10 minutes to properly transition your body back to a rested state.

- Static stretching: Incorporate gentle static stretches, holding each stretch for 20-30 seconds, to release muscle tension and promote flexibility.

- Breathwork: Continue with deep, conscious breathing to help your body and mind relax and cool down gradually.

- Hydrate: Drink water to replenish any fluids lost during your practice and support muscle recovery.

- Self-massage: Use a foam roller or massage balls to gently release any remaining tightness or knots in your muscles, improving circulation and reducing the risk of soreness.

- Mindfulness: Take a few moments to check in with your body, acknowledge any areas that may need extra care, and express gratitude for your practice.

Eating For Recovery and Well-being

- Proper hydration is needed for muscle recovery, joint lubrication, and overall bodily function. Aim to drink water consistently throughout the day, and consider incorporating electrolyte-rich beverages like coconut water after particularly strenuous practices.

- Proteins are the building block for muscle repair and growth. Include lean protein sources like chicken, fish, tofu, legumes, and Greek yogurt in your meals and snacks to support tissue healing and muscle recovery.

- Colorful fruits and vegetables are rich in antioxidants, which help combat oxidative stress and inflammation caused by physical exertion. Incorporate a variety of vibrant produce like berries, leafy greens, bell peppers, and sweet potatoes into your diet.

- Whole grains, quinoa, and starchy vegetables like squash and sweet potatoes provide sustained energy and promote muscle glycogen replenishment, aiding in recovery and preventing fatigue.

- Nuts, seeds, avocados, and fatty fish like salmon are excellent sources of anti-inflammatory omega-3 fatty acids, which can help reduce muscle soreness and joint pain.

- Consume a balanced meal or snack containing protein, carbs, and healthy fats within 30-60 minutes after your practice to kickstart the recovery process and replenish depleted energy stores.

- Consult with a healthcare professional about incorporating supplements like protein powder, BCAAs (branched-chain amino acids), or tart cherry juice to support muscle repair and reduce inflammation, especially if you struggle to meet your nutritional needs through diet alone.

- Be aware of how your body responds to different foods and adjust your diet accordingly. Every individual has unique nutritional needs and preferences.

I know that when it comes to weight loss a lot of us really struggle with the food part, so, here are a few reminders for you that you can come back to when your mind goes back to an unhealthy place.

1. Food is not the enemy. Even if you missed your practice today, you still deserve to eat. We don't work out to earn our food. We move our bodies because deep down, our future selves are whispering, "Please, do this for me. Keep going."

2. Nourishing yourself is an act of respect, not punishment. Food gives you life - quite literally, so approach each meal as a loving opportunity to refuel your amazing body.

3. Progress is the subtle shift, not the blinding transformation. Your relationship with food is an unwinding path, so celebrate each small step forward. Perfection is a fantasy, but you? You're deliciously real.

4. Mindful eating is a sacred pause. It's slowing down to taste life's flavors, feeling each crunch, and savoring your body's cues of satisfaction. It's making peace with the plate.

5. Toss those labels of "good" and "bad" from your inner dialogue, honey. Food is just food until we moralize it with judgments that lead nowhere.

6. Emotional eating has embraced us all at times. Rather than beating yourself up, get curious. What's feeding that hunger within?

7. Let water be your steady companion, keeping your precious body hydrated and happy as you navigate each day's adventures.

8. Movement matters because you matter. Somatic yoga, strolls, stretches - it's all

vital in honoring your extraordinary vessel.

9. You wouldn't speak those cruel words to a friend, so why do you say them to yourself? Self-compassion is the ultimate revolution.

10. The real nourishment is in the journey itself. So grab life with both hands, taking delicious bites out of every moment, taste, and experience.

Chapter Four

Is 10 Minutes Enough?

All or nothing thinking, I don't think that's just a me thing alone. I think it's an all-of-us kind of thing. So many of us carry this burden of believing that we have to go big or go home for there to be any real impact or difference. We get trapped in this mindset that if we can't devote hours upon hours to something, it's not even worth trying.

But here's the truth, one I've had to remind myself of time and again—those small steps we so easily dismiss? They're powerful beyond measure. Letting our progress build up from one tiny, consistent action to the next is not just okay, it might be the most sustainable, transformative way to create lasting change. I was always convinced that I needed to carve out these huge blocks of time every day to "do it right." But between work, family, and all the other demands of life, those lofty goals just left me feeling like a failure before I even began. It was only when I permitted myself to start with just 10 minutes a day that everything shifted.

Those 10 mindful, intentional minutes were my anchor in the storm. They became stepping stones that gave me the confidence and momentum to gradually weave the practice more fully into my life. And you know what? A year later, I looked back in awe at how those "insignificant" 10 minutes had compounded into something profound and life-changing.

Small is indeed mighty, whether it's 10 minutes of somatic yoga or any other positive habit, those modest daily actions are how revolutions begin from within. Sustainable growth starts with the courage to start small and let the miracle of momentum work its magic.

Understanding Time Constraints

Modern lifestyles and expectations can mean we often find ourselves pulled in a million different directions at once. Our lives are a dance between the demands of our careers, the needs of our families, and the unspoken obligations of maintaining an active social circle. During this constant juggling act, carving out time solely for ourselves can feel like an impossible luxury.

In the workplace, we're expected to be high-achievers, constantly proving our worth and dedication. The pressure to excel, meet deadlines, and navigate office politics can be all-consuming, leaving little mental or physical energy for much else.

Then there's the beautiful chaos of family life: tending to the needs of young children, caring for aging parents, and simply managing a household; the roles we play as nurturers, coordinators, and emotional anchors are endless. The idea of "me time" often gets buried beneath a mountain of to-do lists and the relentless demands of keeping it all together.

And let's not forget the way society conditions us to be the "connectors" – the ones who foster and maintain our social circles, plan gatherings, and ensure that the intricate web of relationships remains intact. This invisible labor, while rewarding, can also be draining, leaving us with little bandwidth for self-care.

In between all of these concurrent responsibilities, finding even a pocket of time to devote to our well-being can feel like a monumental challenge. The guilt of "taking" that time for ourselves, of seemingly neglecting our other roles, can be a powerful deterrent. It's precisely because we wear so many hats and give so much of ourselves to others that we must prioritize self-care.. These mindful moments of reconnecting with our bodies, quieting our minds, and tending to our own needs are not just luxuries, they're necessities. They're what allow us to replenish our reserves, find our center, and show up more fully in all the other areas of our lives.

Micro Practices

For those of us strapped for time, the concept of "micro-practices" can be a game-changer in making space for self-care activities like somatic yoga.

Micro-practices are short, intentional moments of mindfulness and movement that can be seamlessly woven into our daily routines. They're the antidote to the "all or nothing" mentality, proving that even a few minutes of focused practice can have a profound impact. Instead of feeling like you need to carve out an hour or more for a full somatic yoga session, you could try a micro-practice of a few simple movements and breathwork while waiting for your morning coffee to brew. Gently roll your shoulders, stretch your neck from side to side, and take a few deep, conscious breaths–all in the span of two or three minutes.

Another example could be using your commute as an opportunity for a micro-practice. While stopped at a red light or waiting for the train, you could do some subtle spinal rotations in your seat, engaging your core and releasing any tension you might be holding in your back. Even something as simple as setting a reminder to take a one-minute "mindful pause" every few hours can be very beneficial. During this pause, you could close your eyes, place a hand on your belly, and focus on the sensation of your breath moving in and out. This short break can help you re-center and return to your tasks with a refreshed perspective.

The beauty of micro-practices is that they can be tailored to fit seamlessly into the nooks and crannies of your day. Perhaps you could spend two minutes doing some gentle neck stretches while your dinner is in the microwave, or take a few calming breaths and engage your core muscles while brushing your teeth.

These bite-sized moments of mindful movement and breathwork may seem insignificant on their own, but when consistently practiced, they can have a cumulative effect on your overall well-being. They're like tiny seeds you're planting throughout your day, which can eventually blossom into a more grounded, centered, and embodied way of being. Micro-practices remind us that self-care doesn't have to be an all-or-nothing thing. When we consciously reframe our perspective and embrace these small, achievable moments, we can gradually cultivate a deeper mind-body connection and a sense of inner peace, even during our busiest days.

The Benefits of Shorter Sessions

Easy does it, that's the one thing that we have established. While the idea of an hour-long somatic yoga session may seem like the ideal, the reality is that shorter, more frequent practices can be just as beneficial, if not more so. Here are some key advantages to embracing these bite-sized sessions:

- Consistency: It's often easier to commit to 10 or 15 minutes a day than to try and carve out a large chunk of time. This consistency, even in small doses, can lead to better habit formation and long-term results.

- Reduced Overwhelm: An entire hour can feel daunting, especially for beginners or those with busy schedules. Shorter sessions feel more manageable and less intimidating, making it easier to stick with the practice.

- Mindfulness: Brief sessions encourage you to be fully present for the entire duration, rather than allowing your mind to wander during a longer practice. This focused mindfulness can deepen the mind-body connection.

- Flexibility: With micro-practices, you can seamlessly integrate somatic yoga into your day whenever you have a few spare minutes – whether it's first thing in the morning, on your lunch break, or right before bed.

- Sustained Energy: Instead of hitting a wall after an intense hour-long session, shorter practices provide an energizing boost without leaving you drained or fatigued.

- Progress Over Perfection: Removing the pressure to complete a full, lengthy routine allows you to focus on the process and enjoy the journey, rather than fixating on an idealized end goal.

The Principles of Effective Short Practices

While the idea of longer sessions may seem more impactful, the truth is that quality trumps quantity, it is not the duration, but the intention, focus, and mindfulness you bring to each practice that matters no matter how brief. Prioritizing these core principles, even if it's a 10-15 minute session can be incredibly powerful, it's about making sure that you thoughtfully curate each element to create a cohesive, nourishing experience for both body and mind. Let's look at what these principles are

Intention: You have to be grounded and there has to be a purpose for your practice, be it a specific area of tension you'd like to release, an emotion you'd like to process, or simply a commitment to being fully present. Clearly defining your intention helps guide the rest of your session.

- Breath Awareness: this is the heartbeat of any somatic practice. You need to be attuned to your natural breathing pattern, then explore different techniques like diaphragmatic breathing, lengthened exhales, or alternate nostril breathing. This oxygenates the body and brings your awareness inward.

- Gentle Movement: You don't have to focus on the whole idea of "no pain", make your movements mindful and focus on the postures that feel intuitive and nourishing for your body at that moment. This could be simple spinal rotations, neck stretches, or any posture that encourages you to tune into bodily sensations, it's all a matter of moving with intention and presence.

- Body Scanning: Take a few moments to mentally scan through each area of your body, noticing any sensations of tension, relaxation, or areas that need extra care. This cultivates proprioception (awareness of your body in space) and allows you to adjust your practice accordingly.

- Focused Attention: Don't try to cram in too many elements, choose one area of focus for your shorter session, like a specific area of the body (e.g., hips, shoulders), an emotional quality (e.g., releasing anxiety), or a universal principle (e.g., cultivating self-compassion). Maintain your attention on this intention throughout the practice.

- Mindful Transition: As you approach the end of your session, take a few moments to reconnect with your breath and your physical sensations. Notice any shifts in your body, mind, or emotional state. This mindful transition helps integrate the benefits of your practice.

- Gratitude and Affirmation: It's always good to end off the session with a proclamation of thanks, and offer a positive affirmation that resonates with your intention. It is a seemingly simple practice that can have such an incredibly uplifting effect.

Allow yourself to be as slow as you want to, it's not about how long you go, but ultimately about what you get out of the whole session.

Balancing Short and Longer Sessions

I know that we've talked a lot about going slowly, but there are also immense benefits to incorporating longer sessions; you have to find a way to get to a point of equilibrium between the two, this is why:

- Longer sessions (30-60 minutes) allow you to get into the nuances of somatic exploration, you get to have more time to slow down, explore subtle movements and sensations, and peel back layers of physical and emotional tension.

- Over time our bodies accumulate stress, anxiety, and stuck, so while shorter practices help manage daily tensions, lengthier sessions create space for a more cathartic release. You get to tap into emotions, memories, or physical blockages arising that need to be fully processed and integrated.

- Extended periods of mindful movement and breathwork can have an incredibly calming effect on the nervous system, helping us to counteract the effects of chronic stress. This regulation is what makes us more resilient, focused, and healthy overall

- Dedicating a larger window of uninterrupted time reinforces your commitment and sends a powerful message to yourself and others that nurturing your mind-body is a priority, not just an afterthought.

- Longer sessions allow for more organic, unstructured exploration. Your intuition starts to lead you and you're braver to try new movements, postures, or breathwork techniques that feel particularly nourishing at that moment. This freedom to follow your body's wisdom deepens self-trust.

- Incorporating a range of practice lengths acts as a form of cross-training. Shorter sessions build consistency and integrate somatic principles into daily life, while extended periods allow for a different type of focus and immersion. Varying the stimulus in this way keeps your practice fresh and engaging.

So just aim to strike a balance that works for your lifestyle, energy levels, and needs. Perhaps most days include a short 10-20 minute practice, with one or two longer 45-60 minute windows each week. This equilibrium allows you to reap the multitude of benefits that both micro-practices and more immersive sessions have to offer.

Chapter Five

Somatic Yoga 50 Illustrated Poses

We're finally at the good stuff - the core of this book and the reason you picked it up in the first place. In the previous chapters, we've covered the principles and philosophy behind somatic yoga, the mind-body connection, and how this approach can facilitate weight loss in a healthy, sustainable manner, but now, it's time to dive into the practical application.

This chapter is a comprehensive guide to 50 carefully curated somatic yoga poses, each one designed to engage your entire being. These postures are not just physical exercises; they are movements that cultivate awareness, presence, and a deep connection with your innermost self.

Each pose is meticulously illustrated, accompanied by step-by-step instructions to ensure proper alignment and execution. Whether you're a seasoned yogi or a complete beginner, these illustrations will serve as your visual aid, enabling you to practice with confidence and precision.

Standing Poses

Standing poses form the foundation of many yoga practices, and somatic yoga is no exception. These postures are designed to cultivate strength, stability, and a sense of grounding within the body. By firmly rooting yourself into the earth, you'll establish a solid base from which to explore the subtleties of movement and breath.

Standing poses are particularly beneficial for cultivating body awareness, improving posture, and toning the muscles of the legs, core, and back. As you practice these poses, you'll learn to engage your entire body, from the soles of your feet to the crown of your head, fostering a heightened sense of integration and presence.

In this section, we'll explore a variety of standing poses, each pose will be accompanied by clear instructions and illustrations, guiding you through the proper alignment and engagement of the muscles involved.

Mountain Pose

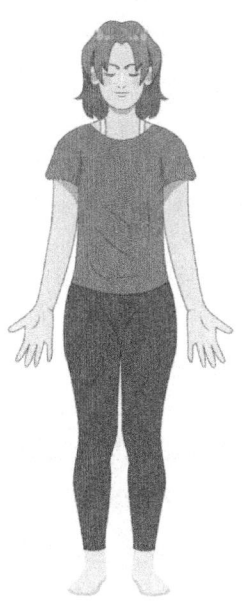

Mountain Pose (Tadasana) is a fundamental yoga posture that serves as the foundation for many other poses. It involves standing tall with feet rooted into the ground, legs engaged, spine elongated, shoulders relaxed, and a sense of stability and strength emanating from the body. This pose helps improve posture, balance, and awareness of alignment, making it an excellent starting point for a yoga practice.

1. Stand tall with your feet hip-width apart, toes pointing forward.

2. Engage your thigh muscles, lift your kneecaps, and tuck your tailbone slightly to align your pelvis.

3. Roll your shoulders back and down, extending your arms alongside your body with palms facing forward.

4. Lengthen your spine by lifting through the crown of your head and grounding through your feet.

5. Relax your face and jaw, and gaze softly ahead, finding a sense of calm and focus.

6. Breathe deeply and evenly, feeling rooted like a mountain, stable and unwavering.

Forward Fold

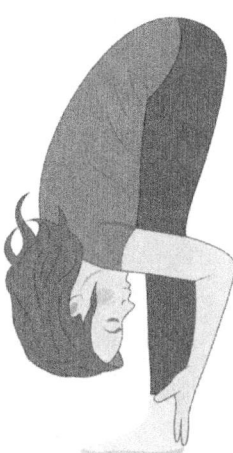

Forward Fold, also known as Uttanasana in yoga, is a calming pose that stretches the entire back body, including the spine, hamstrings, and calves. It promotes relaxation, releases tension, and can help improve digestion and relieve stress. Forward Fold is often practiced to cultivate a sense of surrender and introspection, allowing practitioners to let go of physical and mental burdens.

1. Start in mountain pose

2. Exhale as you hinge at the hips, folding forward from the waist.

3. Keep your spine long as you bend your knees slightly to protect your lower back.

4. Let your head and neck relax, allowing your arms to hang down towards the floor or grabbing opposite elbows.

5. Engage your quadriceps to gently straighten your legs and deepen the stretch in the hamstrings.

6. Breathe deeply and hold the pose for several breaths, feeling the release and lengthening in the back body.

Warrior I

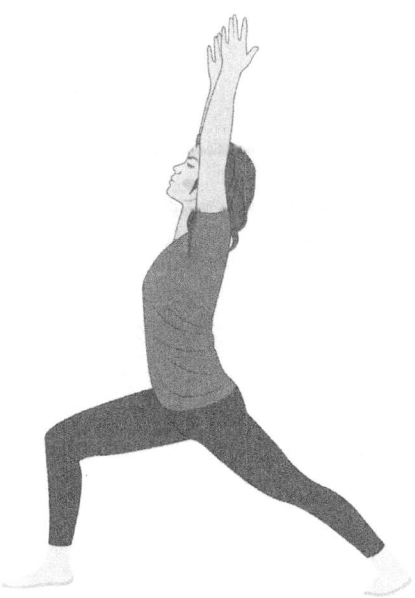

Warrior I, or Virabhadrasana I, is designed to build strength in the legs, opens the hips, and stretches the chest and shoulders. This pose embodies qualities of strength, focus, and determination, helping practitioners cultivate courage and inner resilience.

1. At the top of your mat, position yourself in a mountain pose

2. Step your right foot back about 3-4 feet, keeping your front foot pointing forward and your back foot at a 45-degree angle.

3. Bend your front knee to a 90-degree angle, ensuring it aligns with your ankle.

4. Ground down through the outer edge of your back foot and press the inner thigh of your back leg.

5. Square your hips towards the front of the mat and lift your arms overhead, palms facing each other or hands in prayer position.

6. Lift your chest, lengthen your spine, and gaze forward or up towards your hands.

7. Remain here for several breaths, allowing yourself to feel strong and energized throughout your body.

Warrior II

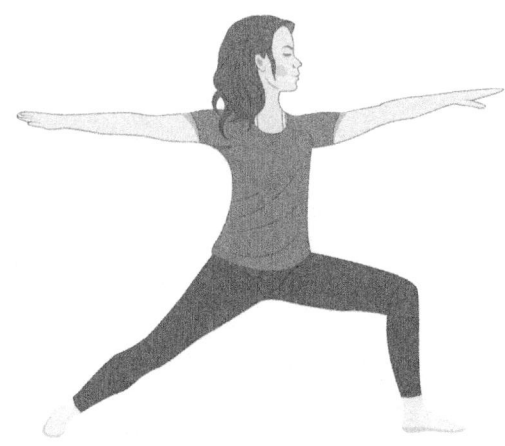

Warrior II is a dynamic yoga pose that strengthens the legs, opens the hips, and improves focus and stamina. This pose embodies qualities of grace, stability, and determination, helping practitioners cultivate inner strength and resilience.

1. Mountain pose is going to be the starting point

2. Step your right foot back about 3-4 feet, keeping your front foot pointing forward and your back foot parallel to the back edge of the mat.

3. Bend your front knee to a 90-degree angle, ensuring it aligns with your ankle.

4. Extend your arms out to the sides at shoulder height, palms facing down.

5. Square your hips towards the side of the mat and gaze over your front fingertips.

6. Keep your shoulders relaxed, chest open, and spine long.

7. Engage your core and leg muscles, grounding down through the outer edge of your back foot.

8. Hold this for a couple of breaths, feeling the strength and determination of a warrior.

Extended Side Angle Pose

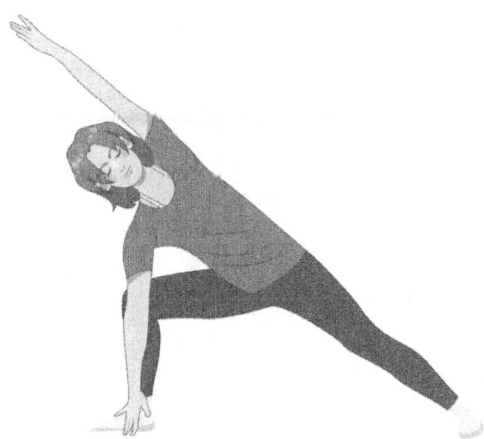

Extended Side Angle Pose, or Utthita Parsvakonasana, is a dynamic yoga pose that strengthens the legs, stretches the side body, and improves balance and focus. This pose cultivates qualities of openness, stability, and expansion, helping practitioners find strength and length in the body.

1. You will start in Warrior II on your right side, with your right knee bent at a 90-degree angle and your arms extended out.

2. Lower your right forearm to your right thigh or the outside of your right foot.

3. Extend your left arm overhead, creating a straight line from your left heel to your fingertips.

4. Keep your chest open, shoulders relaxed, and gaze towards your left fingertips.

5. Engage your core and leg muscles, pressing firmly into the outer edge of your back foot.

6. Lengthen through the side body, feeling a stretch from your left heel to your fingertips.

7. Hold the pose for several breaths, maintaining stability and openness in the body.

Tree Pose

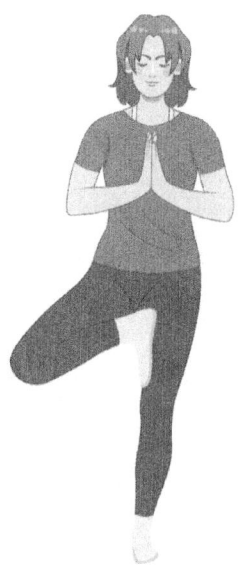

Tree Pose, or Vrksasana, is a balancing yoga pose that strengthens the legs, improves focus and concentration, and promotes stability and grounding. This pose embodies qualities of balance, grace, and rootedness, helping practitioners find inner peace and stability.

1. Start with your feet hip-width apart and arms by your sides.
2. Move your weight onto your left foot and lift your right foot off the ground.
3. Place the sole of your right foot on your inner left thigh, calf, or ankle, avoiding the knee.
4. Press your foot into your leg and your leg back into your foot for stability.
5. Bring your hands to a prayer position at your heart or extend them overhead.
6. Find a focal point to help with balance and keep your gaze soft.
7. Engage your core, lengthen your spine, and breathe deeply.
8. Hold the pose for several breaths, then switch sides.

Chair Pose

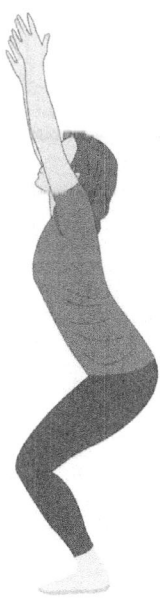

Chair Pose, or Utkatasana, is a strengthening yoga pose that targets the legs, core, and glutes while improving balance and focus. This pose embodies qualities of strength, determination, and resilience, helping practitioners build physical and mental endurance.

1. Place your hands on your hips with your feet hip-width apart.

2. Inhale as you raise your arms overhead, palms facing each other or touching.

3. Exhale and bend your knees, as if sitting back into an imaginary chair.

4. Keep your weight in your heels, knees behind your toes, and thighs parallel to the floor.

5. Engage your core, lengthen your spine, and relax your shoulders away from your ears.

6. Gaze forward or slightly up, finding a focal point for balance.

7. Hold the pose for several breaths, feeling the strength and heat building in your lower body.

Crescent Lunge Pose

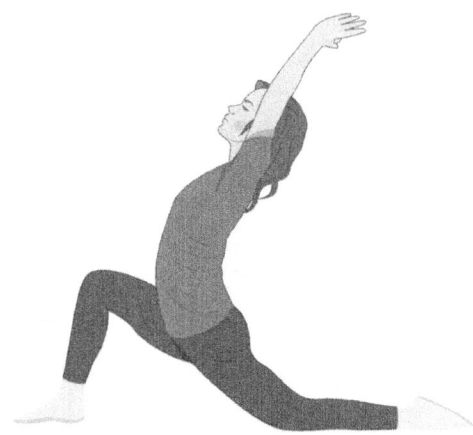

Crescent Lunge or High Lunge strengthens the legs, opens the hips, and stretches the hip flexors and quadriceps. It embodies qualities of strength, balance, and expansion, helping practitioners cultivate energy and vitality.

1. Stand upright at the top of your mat.//
2. Step your right foot back into a lunge position, keeping your right heel lifted and toes grounded.
3. Bend your left knee to a 90-degree angle, ensuring it aligns with your ankle.
4. Keep your right leg straight and engaged, pressing back through your right heel.
5. Lift your arms overhead, palms facing each other, or hands in prayer position.
6. Engage your core, lengthen your spine, and relax your shoulders down.
7. Gaze forward or slightly up, finding a focal point for balance.
8. Keep holding the pose for 5 breaths, feeling the strength and openness in your body.

Half Moon Pose

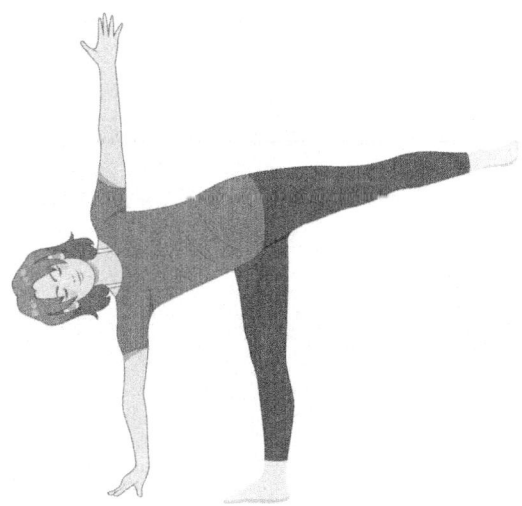

Half Moon Pose, or Ardha Chandrasana, is a balancing yoga pose that strengthens the legs, and core, and improves coordination and focus. This pose involves balancing on one leg while extending the other leg and arm towards the sky, creating a crescent shape with the body. It helps improve balance, stability, and concentration.

1. Stand at the top of your mat.

2. Carry your weight onto your right foot and extend your left leg back, keeping it parallel to the floor.

3. Place your right hand on the mat or a block under your right shoulder for support.

4. Engage your core and lift your left arm towards the sky, stacking your shoulders and hips.

5. Open your chest towards the side and gaze up towards your left fingertips for balance.

6. Keep your standing leg strong and maintain a straight line from your left heel to your fingertips.

7. Hold the pose for several breaths, then gently release and switch sides.

Eagle Pose

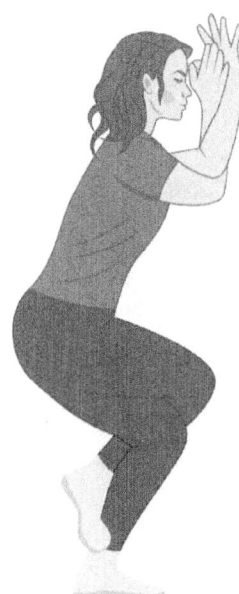

The Eagle Pose (Garudasana) is a standing balancing pose where one leg is crossed over the other leg, and the arms are wrapped around each other in front of the body, mimicking the posture of an eagle, it aims to strengthen the legs, opens the shoulders, and improves focus and concentration.

1. Stand with your feet hip-width apart.
2. Bend your knees slightly and lift your left leg, crossing it over your right thigh.
3. Wrap your left foot around your right calf if possible.
4. Extend your arms out to the sides, then cross your right arm under your left arm at the elbows.
5. Bring your palms together, or press the backs of your hands together.
6. Sink into a seated position, keeping your chest lifted and shoulders relaxed.
7. Gaze softly at a point in front of you to help with balance.
8. keep this way for about 4 breaths, then unwind and switch sides.

Seated Poses

Seated poses, also known as seated asanas, are a big part of any well-rounded yoga practice. While standing poses challenge our balance, strength, and stamina, seated poses offer a different set of benefits that complement the practice as a whole.

They are also very accessible because they give a stable base, allowing you to focus your attention inward and cultivate a deeper sense of body awareness and mindfulness. Whether you're a beginner or an experienced yogi, seated poses offer a gentle way to stretch, lengthen, and realign the body. These grounded postures not only encourage physical flexibility but also promote mental calmness and emotional equilibrium. By rooting the body to the earth, seated poses create a sense of stability and groundedness, which can help quiet the mind and cultivate a meditative state.

Seated poses are often used as preparatory or counterposing asanas, helping to warm up the body for more advanced postures or providing a restorative counterpart to more intense practices, you can also modify these to your liking, adapting them to your level of experience.

Seated Forward Fold (Paschimottanasana)

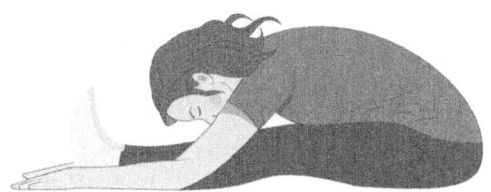

The Seated Forward Fold, or Paschimottanasana, is a seated forward bending pose that stretches the entire back of the body, including the hamstrings, calves, and lower back.

1. Start off in a seated position with your legs extended in front of you, keeping your spine straight and your toes pointing upwards.

2. Breathe deeply, elongating your spine, and exhale while folding forward from your hips, not your waist. Keep your legs firmly pressed into the floor.

3. Reach forward and grab your big toes with your index and middle fingers. If you cannot reach your toes, loop a strap or towel around the soles of your feet to assist you.

4. Inhale and lengthen your spine, then exhale and fold deeper, walking your hands down your legs as far as possible while keeping your legs straight.

5. Rest your torso on your thighs, bringing your forehead as close to your knees as you comfortably can. Relax your neck and shoulders.

6. Hold the pose, breathing deeply through your nose. With each exhalation, fold a little deeper.

7. To release, inhale and slowly roll up to a seated position, vertebra by vertebra.

Butterfly Pose (Baddha Konasana)

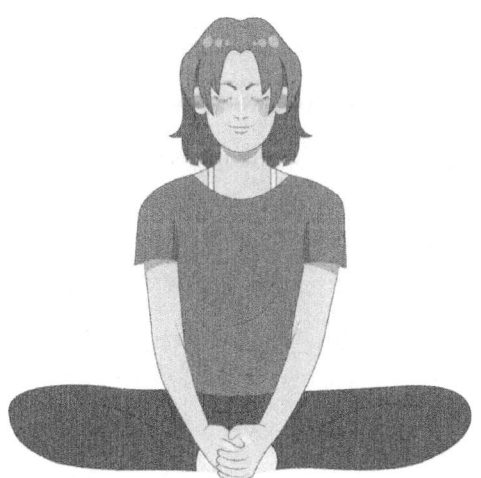

Butterfly Pose is a seated hip opener that stretches the inner thighs, groin, and knees. It can increase hip mobility and flexibility.

1. Sit with your spine straight and legs extended in front of you.

2. Bend your knees and bring the soles of your feet together, allowing your knees to drop towards the floor. Your heels should be as close to your pelvis as possible.

3. Grab your feet or ankles with your hands. Gently pull your heels closer to your body while pressing your knees towards the floor with your elbows.

4. Keeping your spine erect, begin to hinge forward from your hips, walking your hands forward as far as is comfortable. Rest your torso on or towards your thighs.

5. Hold the pose, breathing deeply. With each exhalation, allow your knees to release towards the floor.

6. To intensify the stretch, gently push your knees towards the floor with your elbows on each inhalation.

7. To release, inhale and slowly lift your torso upright using your abdominal muscles. Straighten your legs.

Seated Twist (Ardha Matsyendrasana)

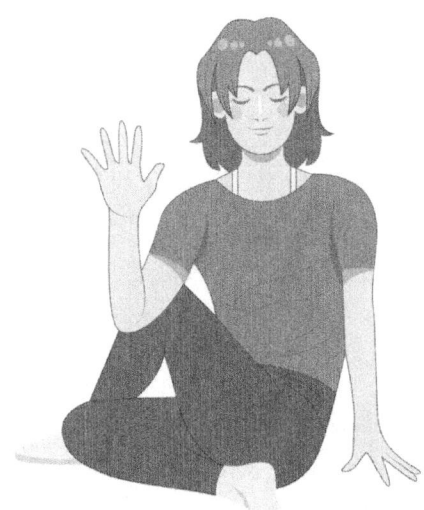

The Seated Twist, or Ardha Matsyendrasana, is a deep twisting pose that provides an intense spiral stretch for the spine, shoulders, and hips. This deep twisting pose not only improves spinal mobility and flexibility but also massages the abdominal organs, aiding digestion and detoxification. It can also help relieve lower back pain and improve overall posture.

1. Extend your legs in front of you. Bend your left knee and bring your left foot under your right knee, keeping your right leg extended.

2. Inhale and elongate your spine. As you exhale, twist your upper body towards your right, placing your left hand on the floor behind you and your right hand on your right knee or thigh.

3. Keep both sitting bones grounded, and twist from the base of your spine. With each inhalation, lengthen your spine, and with each exhalation, twist a little deeper.

4. Turn your head to look over your right shoulder, but avoid straining your neck. Engage your abdominal muscles to deepen the twist.

5. Hold the pose for several breaths, breathing deeply into the twist. Switch sides, repeating the instructions for the opposite side.

Boat Pose (Navasana)

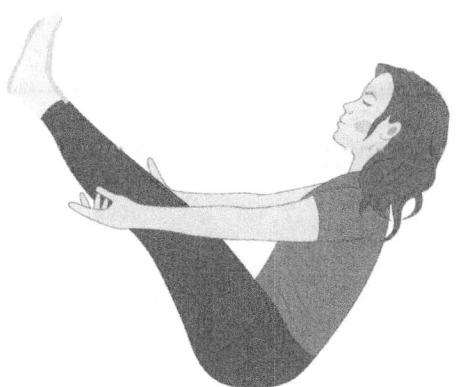

The Boat Pose, or Navasana, is a seated balancing pose that engages the entire body, from the core muscles to the arms and legs. It is a great core strengthener that also tones the abdominal muscles, hip flexors, and spine. It improves balance, concentration, and mental focus while challenging your endurance and determination.

1. Sit with your legs outstretched in front of you, feet together, and arms by your sides.

2. breathe in deeply, engaging your abdominal muscles and leaning back slightly, balancing on your sitting bones.

3. As you exhale, lift your legs off the floor, keeping them straight and together, forming a "V" shape with your body. Your torso should be leaning back at a 45-degree angle, with your arms extended parallel to the floor.

4. Engage your core muscles by drawing your navel towards your spine and squeezing your inner thighs together. Keep your gaze focused straight ahead to maintain balance.

5. For an added challenge, extend your arms alongside your legs, reaching towards your feet or shins.

6. Hold the pose, breathing deeply and evenly through your nose. Engage your core muscles with each exhalation to maintain the "V" shape.

7. To release, exhale and slowly lower your legs and torso back to the starting seated position.

Wide-Legged Forward Fold (Upavistha Konasana)

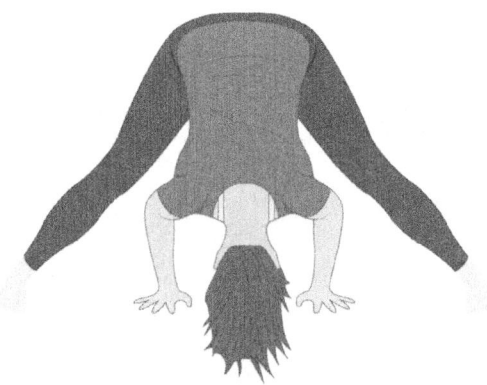

The Wide-Legged Forward Fold, or Upavistha Konasana, is a seated forward bend that provides an intense stretch for the inner thighs, hamstrings, and lower back. This pose is particularly beneficial for improving flexibility and promoting relaxation.

1. Sit with your as wide apart as possible, creating a straight line with your inner thighs and feet.

2. Flex your feet, actively engaging your quadriceps and the muscles in your thighs.

3. Inhale deeply, elongating your spine, and exhale while folding forward from your hips, not your lower back. Keep your torso long and your spine straight as you hinge forward.

4. Walk your hands forward as far as possible, placing them on the floor in front of you or holding onto your big toes or a strap if you cannot reach the floor.

5. Every time you breathe in, fold deeper into the pose, releasing tension in your lower back and hamstrings. Allow your head to hang heavy, releasing any remaining tension in your neck and shoulders.

6. Hold the pose for several breaths, breathing deeply into the areas that feel tight or restricted.

7. To release, inhale and slowly roll up to a seated position, vertebra by vertebra, leading with your chest.

Seated Wide-Legged Straddle (Upavistha Konasana)

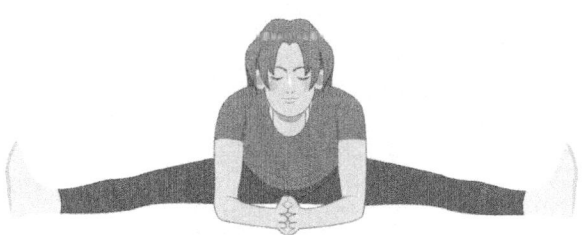

The Seated Wide-Legged Straddle is a seated forward bend that provides an intense stretch for the inner thighs, hamstrings, and lower back which is an excellent way to improve flexibility and promote relaxation.

1. Sit with your legs straight, creating a straight line with your inner thighs and feet. Your legs should be as wide apart as possible.

2. Flex your feet, actively engaging your quadriceps and the muscles in your thighs.

3. Inhale deeply, lengthening your spine, and as you exhale, hinge forward from your hips, not your lower back. Keep your torso long and your spine straight as you fold forward.

4. Walk your hands forward as far as possible, placing them on the floor in front of you or holding onto your big toes or a strap if you cannot reach the floor.

5. With each exhalation, fold deeper into the pose, releasing tension in your lower back, hamstrings, and inner thighs. Allow your head to hang heavy, releasing any remaining tension in your neck and shoulders.

6. Hold the pose for several breaths, breathing deeply into the areas that feel tight or restricted.

7. To release, inhale and slowly roll up to a seated position, vertebra by vertebra, leading with your chest.

Half Lord of the Fishes Pose (Ardha Matsyendrasana)

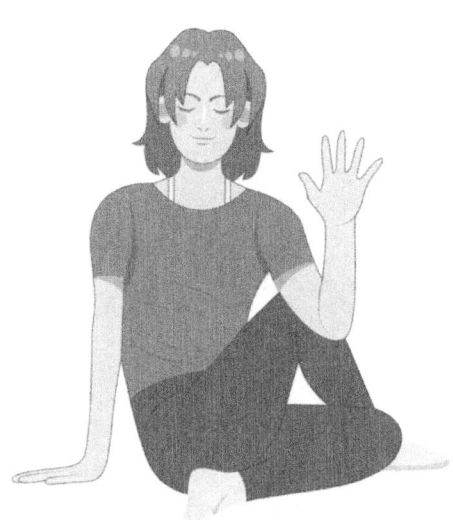

Ardha Matsyendrasana, or Half Lord of the Fishes Pose, is a seated spinal twist that provides an intense stretch for the back, shoulders, and hips. You can use this pose to improve spinal mobility and flexibility while massaging the abdominal organs, aiding digestion and detoxification. It can also help relieve lower back pain and improve overall posture.

1. Stretch your legs in front of you, bend your right knee, and cross it over your left leg, placing your right foot flat on the floor beside your left knee.

2. Breathe in and elongate your spine. As you exhale, twist your upper body towards your right, placing your left hand on the floor behind you and your right hand on the floor beside your right hip.

3. Keep both sitting bones grounded, and twist from the base of your spine. With each inhalation, lengthen your spine, and with each exhalation, twist a little deeper.

4. Turn your head to look over your right shoulder, but avoid straining your neck. Engage your abdominal muscles to deepen the twist.

5. Hold the pose for several breaths, breathing deeply into the twist. Switch sides, repeating the instructions for the opposite side.

Cow Face Pose (Gomukhasana)

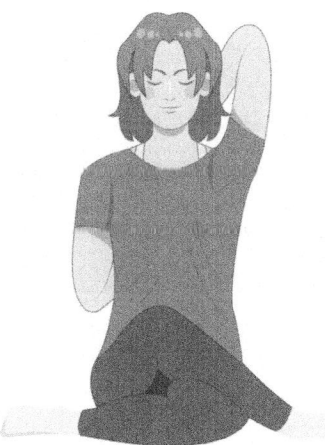

Cow Face Pose (Gomukhasana) is a deep-twisting posture that targets the shoulders, hips, and spine. It's called "Cow Face" because the positioning of the legs and arms resembles the face of a cow.

1. Sit with your legs outstretched in front of you. Bend your knees and bring the soles of your feet together, allowing your knees to release toward the floor – this is the Bound Angle Pose.

2. Stack your right knee on top of your left knee, creating a cross-legged position. Your right ankle should be near your left hip crease.

3. Reach your right arm overhead, and bend your elbow, allowing your hand to rest between your shoulder blades. If possible, bind your fingers together behind your back.

4. Extend your left arm out to the side, parallel to the floor. Bend your elbow and reach your left hand up toward the ceiling, creating a horizontal line with your left arm.

5. On an inhalation, rotate your upper body to the right, moving your left shoulder blade toward your right knee. Your left hand can either reach toward your right foot or remain extended, depending on your flexibility.

6. Hold the pose for several breaths, keeping your spine long and your gaze forward or down.

7. To release, inhale, and slowly unwind, returning to the center.

8. Repeat on the other side, crossing your left knee on top and switching the arm positions.

Seated Forward Bend with Legs Crossed (Paschimottanasana Variation)

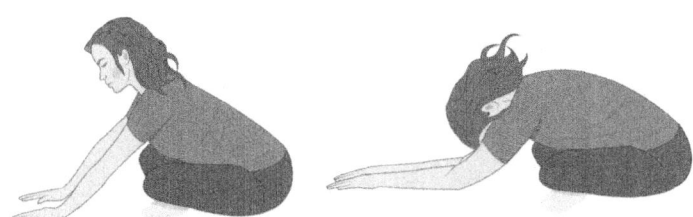

This variation of the Seated Forward Bend, or Paschimottanasana, incorporates a cross-legged seated position, providing a deeper stretch for the hamstrings, calves, and lower back.

1. Sit with both legs extended in front of you, feet together, and spine straight.

2. Cross your right leg over your left, placing your right foot flat on the floor beside your left knee. Then, cross your left leg over your right, stacking your legs one on top of the other.

3. Inhale deeply, elongating your spine, and exhale while folding forward from your hips, not your waist. Keep your legs firmly pressed into the floor.

4. Reach forward and grab your big toes with your index and middle fingers. If you cannot reach your toes, loop a strap or towel around the soles of your feet to assist you.

5. Inhale and lengthen your spine, then exhale and fold deeper, walking your hands down your legs as far as possible while keeping your legs crossed.

6. Rest your torso on your thighs, bringing your forehead as close to your legs as you comfortably can. Relax your neck and shoulders.

7. Hold the pose, breathing deeply through your nose. With each exhalation, fold a little deeper.

8. To release, inhale and slowly roll up to a seated position, vertebra by vertebra.

Seated Spinal Twist (Marichyasana)

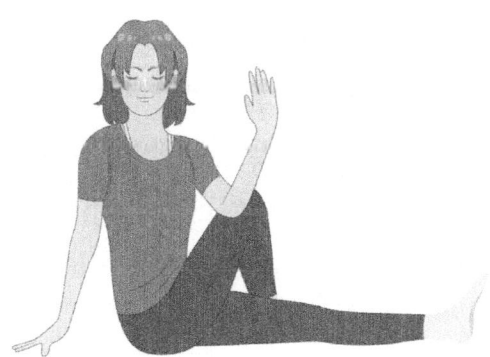

The Seated Spinal Twist, or Marichyasana, is a deep twisting pose that provides an intense spiral stretch for the spine, shoulders, and hips. This pose is excellent for improving spinal mobility, stimulating the abdominal organs, and relieving lower back tightness.

1. Sit with outstretched legs, bend your right knee, and bring your right foot across your left thigh, placing it flat on the floor beside your left knee.

2. Elongate your spine. As you exhale, twist your upper body towards your right, hooking your left elbow on the outside of your right knee or thigh.

3. Place your right hand on the floor behind you for support, and lengthen your spine with each inhalation.

4. With each exhalation, twist deeper, using your left elbow to gently encourage the twist. Turn your head to look over your right shoulder, but avoid straining your neck.

5. Hold the pose for several breaths, breathing deeply into the twist. Engage your abdominal muscles to deepen the twist further.

6. To release, inhale, and unwind your body, bringing your right foot back to the center. Repeat on the opposite side.

Supine Poses

Supine Poses, as the name suggests, are performed while lying on your back. Now, before you start picturing yourself dozing off, let me assure you that these postures are far from passive. They engage your core muscles, open up your hips and chest, and promote a sense of grounding and relaxation that is essential for any well-rounded yoga practice.

From the classic Bridge Pose, which helps strengthen your back and open your heart center, to the delightfully named Happy Baby, which stretches your inner thighs and promotes a playful, childlike spirit, these asanas will leave you feeling refreshed, rejuvenated, and ready to tackle whatever life throws your way.

These poses also offer a wonderful opportunity to cultivate mindfulness and inner peace. While you lie on your mat, you'll learn to tune into your breath, release tension from your body, and perhaps even drift into a blissful state of meditation (don't worry, we'll guide you through it)!

Reclining Bound Angle Pose (Supta Baddha Konasana)

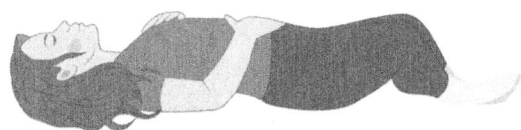

Reclining Bound Angle Pose, also known as Supta Baddha Konasana, is a restorative and hip-opening posture that allows you to relax deeply while gently stretching your inner thighs, groin, and knees.

1. Sit on your mat with your legs extended straight out in front of you. Keep your spine tall.

2. Bend your knees and drop them out to the sides, bringing the soles of your feet together and allowing

your knees to lower towards the floor.

3. With your heels as close to your pelvis as is comfortable, create a diamond or "bound angle" shape with your legs.

4. Lengthen your spine and lean back, lying down on your forearms or back onto the floor if comfortable for your neck.

5. You can place a folded blanket or bolster under your shoulders and head for extra support.

6. Allow your arms to relax out to the sides, palms facing upwards.

7. Release any tension or gripping in your leg muscles and wiggle your sit bones underneath you to create more space in your inner thighs and groin.

8. Breathe deeply into your low belly, allowing your knees to release towards the floor as you relax the soles of your feet together.

9. If having your feet pulled in close causes strain on your knees, slide your heels away from your pelvis until you feel a comfortable stretch.

10. You can place folded blankets or blocks under your thighs for additional support.

11. Stay in the pose for several minutes, breathing into the inner thigh stretch while feeling your spine lengthen along the floor.

12. To release, use your hands to press your knees back together and extend your legs out in front of you.

13. Take a few moments in a simple cross-legged seat to notice the effects of the posture.

Supine Spinal Twist (Supta Matsyendrasana)

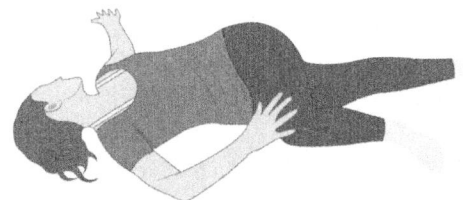

Supine Spinal Twist (Supta Matsyendrasana) is a reclined twisting yoga pose that helps release tension in the lower back and spine. It gently rotates and lengthens the spinal column, improving mobility and flexibility.

1. Lie on your back, legs extended and arms out to the sides in a T-shape.
2. Bend knees and drop them over to the left side, stacking knees and feet.
3. Turn your head to the right and keep your shoulders squared to the floor. Engage core.
4. Optional: Reach your right arm across your body, placing a hand on the outside of your thigh.
5. Press the left outer thigh against the right inner thigh to intensify the twist in the lower back.
6. Take 5-10 deep breaths, releasing into the twist with each exhale.
7. Use your abs to bring your knees back to the center, and extend your legs briefly.
8. Repeat on the other side.
9. Rest in Savasana, noticing effects on the spine.

Happy Baby Pose (Ananda Balasana)

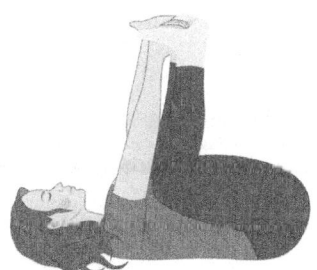

Happy Baby Pose (Ananda Balasana) is a fun and playful hip-opening posture that helps stretch the inner thighs, groin, and lower back. It resembles the positioning of a happy baby, with your feet pulled towards your body while holding the outsides of your feet, creating a big smile-like shape with your legs.

1. Lie down on your back and bring your knees into your chest. Grab the outsides of your feet with your hands.

2. With an inhale, open your knees wider than hip-width apart, letting your knees move towards the floor beside your torso. Your shins should be perpendicular to the floor.

3. Keeping your grip on the outsides of your feet, gently pull your feet down towards the floor behind you, allowing your knees to move towards your armpits.

4. At the same time, use your elbows to push your knees away from your chest, creating more space for your hips and groin. Your ankles should be directly over your knees.

5. Release any tension in your lower back by rocking gently side-to-side. Allow your tailbone to melt into the floor.

6. Breathe deeply into your belly, focusing on the sensation of the inner thigh stretch. You can straighten the arms to intensify the stretch.

7. For a neck release, allow your head to roll from side to side or extend it towards the floor behind you.

8. Hold the pose for 30 seconds to 1 minute, breathing through any sensations of tightness or release.

9. To release, remove your grip from the feet and extend your legs back to the floor with an exhale.

Supine Figure Four Stretch (Supine Pigeon Pose)

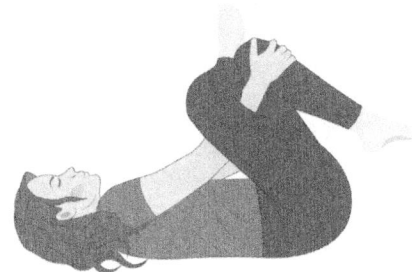

This is a reclined hip-opening stretch where you cross one ankle over the opposite thigh to open up the hips and glutes while lying on your back.

1. Lie down on your back and bend your knees, bringing the soles of your feet to the floor hip-width apart.

2. Cross your right ankle over your left thigh, creating a figure-4 shape with your legs.

3. Thread your hands between your legs and behind your left thigh. Grab the back of your left thigh or calf.

4. With an inhale, draw your left thigh towards your chest, keeping your right foot flexed.

5. Use your hands to pull the left thigh closer, deepening the stretch in your right glute and hip.

6. Keep your head and shoulders planted on the floor throughout the stretch.

7. Take 5-10 deep breaths, feeling the intense but therapeutic stretch in your right hip and glute.

8. To release, remove your hands and slowly lower your left leg back to the floor with an exhale.

9. Repeat on the other side by crossing your left ankle over your right thigh into a figure-4.

10. Grab behind your right thigh and pull it towards your chest to feel the stretch in your left glute/hip.

11. Hold for 5-10 breaths before releasing back to the floor.

12. You can do a few rounds of this pose, allowing your hips to open up further each time.

Legs Up the Wall Pose (Viparita Karani)

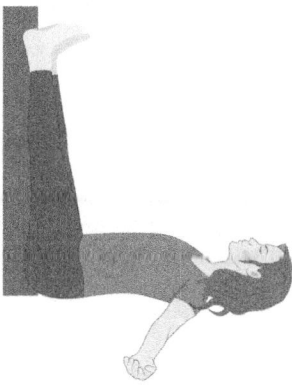

This is an inverted pose where you rest your legs up against a wall, allowing gravity to provide a gentle stretch and release tension in your hamstrings, calves, back, and mind.

1. Position yourself sitting sideways against a wall, with one hip and side of your body touching the wall.

2. Walk your feet up the wall, then rotate your body to lie down on your back, bringing your legs up to rest against the wall.

3. Shift your body so that your sit bones are a few inches away from the wall. Your legs should be straight up the wall.

4. Allow your arms to relax at your sides, palms facing up, or you can place a small pillow under your head/upper back for support.

5. Let your shoulders and head relax towards the floor. Close your eyes if that feels comfortable.

6. Take deep breaths, feeling your spine lengthen with each inhale and the backs of your legs relax with each exhale against the wall.

7. To deepen the stretch in your hamstrings, you can straighten your legs actively or place a strap/belt around the mid-thigh portion of your legs.

8. Stay in this pose for 5-15 minutes, using your breath to fully surrender into the posture.

9. To release, bend your knees and roll over to one side. Use your hands to push yourself back up to a seated position.

10. Take a few moments to orient yourself before standing up from this inverted pose.

Reclining Hand-to-Big-Toe Pose (Supta Padangusthasana)

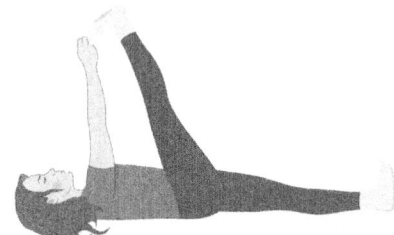

Reclining Hand-to-Big-Toe Pose, also known as Supta Padangusthasana in yoga, is a relaxing and rejuvenating posture that helps stretch the hamstrings, hips, and groins. It also improves balance and focus while promoting a sense of calm.

1. Start by lying on your back on a yoga mat with your legs extended and your arms resting by your sides, palms facing down.

2. Bend your right knee and hug it towards your chest. Keep your left leg extended along the mat, engaging the thigh muscles.

3. Place a yoga strap or a towel around the arch of your right foot. Hold the strap with both hands, keeping your arms extended.

4. On an inhalation, extend your right leg up towards the ceiling, keeping it as straight as possible. You can choose to keep a slight bend in the knee if needed, especially if you feel tightness in the hamstrings.

5. Flex your right foot and press through the heel while keeping the toes pointing towards your face. This helps to deepen the stretch in the calf and hamstring.

6. Relax your shoulders and neck, allowing them to rest comfortably on the mat. Keep both hips grounded and square, avoiding any twisting in the pelvis.

7. Hold the pose for 30 seconds to 1 minute, breathing deeply and evenly. You can gently guide your leg closer to your torso using the strap if you want a deeper stretch.

8. To release the pose, bend your right knee and gently lower the leg back down to the mat. Repeat the same sequence on the other side by switching legs.

9. After completing both sides, you can hug both knees to your chest to release any tension in the lower back.

Reclining Hero Pose (Supta Virasana)

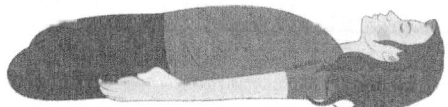

Reclining Hero Pose, also known as Supta Virasana in yoga, is a gentle backbend that stretches the thighs, knees, and ankles while opening the chest and shoulders. It can be a soothing and restorative posture that helps release tension in the front of the body and promotes a sense of calm and relaxation. Practice this pose mindfully and with awareness of your body's limits to fully experience its benefits.

1. Begin by kneeling on the floor with your knees together and your feet slightly wider than hip-width apart. Your toes should be pointing straight back behind you.

2. Slowly lower your hips to the mat, sitting on your heels. If this causes discomfort or strain in your knees, you can place a folded blanket or cushion between your hips and heels for support.

3. From the seated position, gently lower your upper body down to the mat behind you. Use your hands to support yourself as you lean back, keeping your elbows on the floor.

4. Once you are comfortably reclined, extend your arms alongside your body with your palms facing up. You can also place your hands on your abdomen or reach them overhead to increase the stretch in your shoulders.

5. Relax your entire body, allowing your chest to open and your shoulders to soften. Take slow, deep breaths, focusing on expanding the ribcage with each inhale and releasing any tension with each exhale.

6. Stay in Reclining Hero Pose for 1-2 minutes, or longer if it feels comfortable. Be mindful of any sensations in your knees, hips, or lower back, and adjust the pose as needed to ensure you are not experiencing pain.

7. To come out of the pose, engage your core muscles and use your hands to help support yourself as you slowly sit back up. Take a moment to rest in a comfortable seated position before moving on to your next posture.

Reclining Bound Angle Twist (Supta Baddha Konasana Twist)

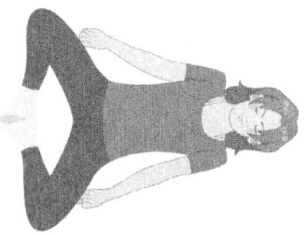

Reclining Bound Angle Twist is a gentle and restorative yoga pose that helps release tension in the spine, hips, and inner thighs while providing a gentle twist to the torso. This pose can help improve flexibility, relieve lower back discomfort, and promote relaxation.

1. Begin by lying on your back on a yoga mat with your legs extended and your arms resting by your sides, palms facing down.

2. Bend your knees and bring the soles of your feet together, allowing your knees to fall out to the sides. This is Bound Angle Pose (Baddha Konasana).

3. Inhale and on an exhale, drop both knees to one side, keeping the soles of your feet together. Your hips and lower back will twist in the direction opposite to where your knees are falling.

4. Extend your arms out to the sides in a T-position, palms facing up, to create a gentle opening in the chest and shoulders.

5. Gently turn your head in the opposite direction of your knees to deepen the twist in the spine. Keep both shoulders grounded on the mat.

6. Close your eyes and relax into the twist, allowing your breath to flow naturally. Feel the stretch along the spine, hips, and inner thighs.

7. Hold the twist for 30 seconds to 1 minute, breathing deeply and evenly. You may deepen the stretch by gently pressing the knees closer to the floor with your hand.

8. On an inhale, slowly return your knees to the center and then exhale as you drop them to the other side, repeating the twist on the opposite side.

9. After completing both sides, bring your knees back to the center and extend your legs out straight to rest in Corpse Pose (Savasana) for a few breaths, allowing your body to integrate the effects of the twist.

Supine Butterfly Stretch (Supta Baddha Konasana Variation)

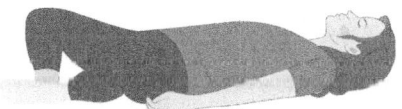

The Supine Butterfly Stretch, also known as Supta Baddha Konasana Variation, is a gentle, reclined posture that targets the inner thighs, groin, and hip area. It is an excellent stretch for improving flexibility and range of motion in these areas, which can be particularly beneficial for individuals seeking to enhance their overall mobility and comfort during physical activities or exercise routines.

Here is a step-by-step explanation of how you perform the Supine Butterfly Stretch

1. Lie down on your back on a flat, comfortable surface like a yoga mat or carpet. Keep your legs extended and your arms by your sides, palms facing down.

2. Bend your knees and bring the soles of your feet together, allowing your knees to fall out to the sides. Your feet should be as close to your groin as possible, depending on your flexibility.

3. Take a few deep breaths, allowing your knees to relax and sink closer to the floor with each exhalation.

4. You can place your hands on your knees or inner thighs and gently press them toward the floor, increasing the stretch in your inner thighs and groin area.

5. Keep your shoulders and head relaxed on the floor, and engage your abdominal muscles to support your lower back.

6. Breathe deeply and hold the pose for several breaths, aiming for 30 seconds to a minute, or as long as comfortable.

7. To release the pose, use your hands to support your knees and bring them back to the center, then extend your legs out in front of you.

8. Repeat the stretch a few times, focusing on your breath and gradually increasing the intensity of the stretch as your body allows.

Reclining Hamstring Stretch (Supta Padangusthasana Variation)

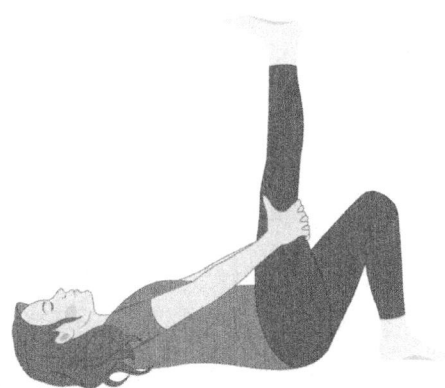

Reclining Hamstring Stretch (Supta Padangusthasana Variation) is a gentle yet effective pose that targets the hamstrings, calves, and lower back. It is a variation of the classic Padangusthasana (Big Toe Pose) but performed in a reclined position, making it more accessible and less demanding on the body. This stretch can help improve flexibility, reduce tension, and promote overall relaxation in the targeted areas.

1. Lie down on your back on a flat, comfortable surface like a yoga mat or carpet. Extend your legs in front of you, keeping them together and your arms by your sides, palms facing down.

2. Bend your right knee and bring it toward your chest, holding the back of your thigh with both hands. Alternatively, you can loop a strap or towel around the ball of your foot to assist in the stretch.

3. Keeping your left leg extended on the floor, inhale and straighten your right leg toward the ceiling, actively engaging your quadriceps.

4. On an exhalation, begin to lower your extended right leg toward the floor, keeping your leg as straight as possible and your quadriceps engaged. Stop when you feel a comfortable stretch in your hamstring.

5. If possible, try to keep both shoulders flat on the floor. If you need more support, you can place a folded blanket or towel under your lower back.

6. Breathe deeply and hold the pose for several breaths, aiming for 30 seconds to a minute, or as long as comfortable.

7. To release the pose, exhale and slowly bend your right knee, bringing it back towards your chest. Lower

your right leg to the floor.

8. Repeat the stretch on the other side, bending your left knee and extending your left leg toward the ceiling.

9. Remember to keep your abdominal muscles engaged to support your lower back and avoid straining your neck by keeping your head relaxed on the floor.

Prone Poses

Prone poses are a category of yoga postures performed while lying on the stomach or front side of the body. These poses are beneficial for stretching the back, shoulders, and chest, as well as strengthening the core and improving spinal alignment.

Backbends (Prone Backbends)

These poses involve arching the back and opening the front of the body, including the chest, abdomen, and hip flexors. Prone backbends can help counteract the effects of prolonged sitting or poor posture, which can lead to a rounded upper back and tight chest muscles. They promote spinal mobility, improve breathing capacity, and can also energize the body by stimulating the nervous system.

Prone Arm and Leg Stretches

These poses involve extending and stretching the arms and legs while lying on the stomach. They can help improve flexibility in the shoulders, hamstrings, and lower back, as well as enhance overall body awareness and control. Prone arm and leg stretches can also relieve tension and promote relaxation in the targeted areas.

Prone Core Strengtheners

These poses engage and strengthen the muscles of the core, including the abdominal muscles, lower back, and obliques. Prone core strengtheners can improve posture, enhance stability, and protect the spine from injury. They can also help develop body awareness and control, which is essential for more advanced yoga poses and physical activities.

Prone poses are generally considered gentler and less intense than standing or inverted poses, making them accessible to a wide range of practitioners, including beginners or those with physical limitations. However, it's still important to practice these poses with proper alignment and mindfulness to avoid strain or injury.

Sphinx Pose (Salamba Bhujangasana)

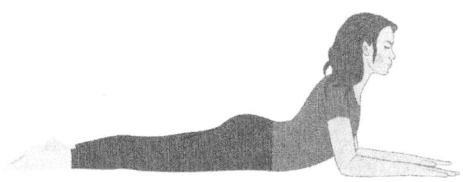

The Sphinx Pose, also known as Salamba Bhujangasana, is a gentle backbend pose that is often used as a preparatory posture for more advanced backbends. It involves lying on the stomach while propping up the upper body with the forearms and elbows. This position creates a gentle arc in the back, opening the chest and stretching the front of the body. The pose is named after the famous Egyptian Sphinx statue, as the posture resembles the reclining sphinx figure with the upper body raised.

1. You will lie on your stomach with your legs extended straight behind you, hip-width apart, and the tops of your feet resting on the floor.

2. Bring your elbows directly under your shoulders, and place your forearms on the floor parallel to each other, forming a straight line from your elbows to your hands.

3. Inhale and press your forearms and hands firmly into the floor, using your back muscles to lift your upper body off the floor. Keep your elbows tucked in close to your body, and engage your abdominal muscles to protect your lower back.

4. As you lift your chest, keep your shoulders relaxed and away from your ears, and gaze forward or slightly upward, but avoid straining your neck.

5. Engage your leg muscles and press the tops of your feet into the floor, creating a gentle backbend through your entire spine.

6. Breathe deeply and hold the pose for several breaths, focusing on lengthening your spine and opening your chest.

7. To release the pose, exhale and slowly lower your upper body back to the floor, keeping your abdominal muscles engaged to protect your lower back.

Cobra Pose (Bhujangasana)

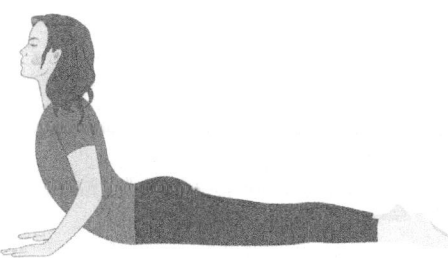

Cobra Pose is a classic backbend asana that targets the spine, abdomen, chest, and shoulders. It is a moderate backbend that can help improve spinal mobility, open the chest and heart area, and invigorate the body.

In this pose, you lie on your stomach with the tops of your feet flat on the floor and your legs together. The upper body is then arched backward, supported by the strength of the back muscles and the hands placed on the floor beside the chest.

1. Lie on your stomach with your legs extended back, the tops of your feet on the floor. Place your hands beside your chest, palms down under your shoulders.

2. Inhale and use your back muscles to gently lift your head, chest, and abdomen off the floor. Keep your navel on the floor, arch your back, and open your chest.

3. Firm the shoulder blades onto your back and look upward, being careful not to strain your neck. You can keep a slight bend in the elbows or straighten the arms, depending on your flexibility.

4. Engage your buttocks and leg muscles to ground the lower body and create a smooth upward arc in your spine.

5. Breathe deeply into the chest and hold the pose for 15-30 seconds, maintaining awareness in your body.

6. To release, exhale and slowly lower your torso to the floor, rolling down from the head to the toes.

You may want to keep the cobra backbend mild, lifting only a few inches off the floor. More advanced practitioners can deepen the backbend by pushing the chest further through and straightening the arms.

Locust Pose (Salabhasana)

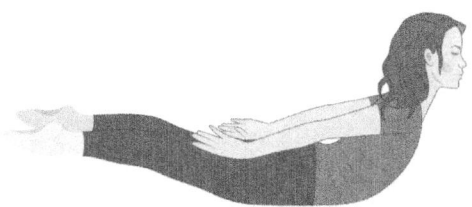

Locust Pose (Salabhasana) is a backbend asana that primarily targets the muscles of the back, buttocks, and legs. It is an excellent exercise for strengthening the core and improving posture.

1. Lie flat on your stomach on a yoga mat or a firm surface. Your legs should be together, and your arms should be at your sides, palms facing down.

2. Inhale deeply, and as you exhale, lift your head, chest, arms, and legs off the floor. Your body should form a gentle arc, with only your lower abdomen and pelvic area remaining on the floor.

3. Engage your back muscles by squeezing your shoulder blades together and reaching your arms back, parallel to the floor. Keep your arms active, with your palms facing downwards.

4. Lift your legs off the floor, keeping them together and straight. Engage your glutes and thigh muscles to support the lift. Avoid arching your lower back excessively.

5. Breathe deeply and hold the pose for 5-10 breaths, or as long as comfortable. Focus on lengthening your body and creating a gentle backbend.

6. To release the pose, exhale and slowly lower your arms, legs, and chest back to the floor. Rest for a few breaths before repeating the pose or moving on to the next asana.

Remember to keep your movements controlled and your core engaged throughout the pose. If you experience any discomfort or strain, modify the pose by lifting your arms and legs only slightly off the floor, or consider using props like blocks or folded blankets for support.

Bow Pose (Dhanurasana)

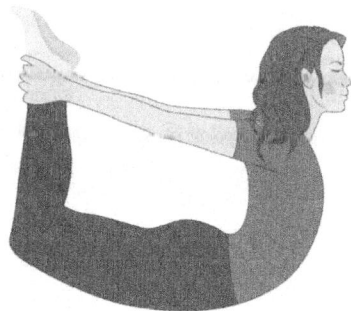

Bow Pose is a deep backbend that stretches the entire front body, including the chest, abdomen, and quadriceps.

1. Lie flat on your stomach with your feet hip-width apart and your arms at your sides.

2. Bend your knees and reach back with your hands to grab the outsides of your ankles.

3. Inhale and lift your heels away from your buttocks while simultaneously lifting your thighs off the floor.

4. Kick your feet into your hands, creating a bow-like shape with your body. Your body should form an arc, with your heels pulling towards your buttocks.

5. Keep your arms parallel to each other and look straight ahead or slightly up.

6. Engage your back muscles and breathe deeply, holding the pose for 5-10 breaths.

7. To release, exhale and slowly lower your legs and upper body back to the floor.

Baby Cobra Pose (Ardha Bhujangasana)

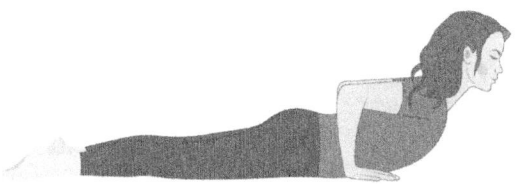

This gentle backbend is an excellent preparatory pose for more advanced back extensions.

1. Lie on your stomach with your legs together and the tops of your feet on the floor.
2. Place your hands beneath your shoulders, with your elbows tucked in close to your body.
3. Inhale and use your back muscles to lift your head, chest, and abdomen off the floor.
4. Keep your navel on the floor and maintain a slight curve in your lower back.
5. Breathe deeply and hold the pose for 5-10 breaths, focusing on lengthening your spine.
6. To release, exhale and slowly lower your body back to the starting position.

Remember to keep your movements controlled and your breathing steady throughout these poses. Modify or use props as needed for comfort and safety.

Crocodile Pose (Makarasana)

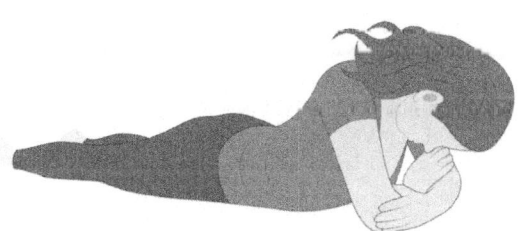

Crocodile Pose is a deep hip opener that also stretches the lower back, shoulders, and chest. It is an intense pose that requires flexibility and should be approached with caution, especially for beginners.

1. Begin in a seated position with your legs extended in front of you, feet together, and spine erect.

2. Bend your knees and bring the soles of your feet together, allowing your knees to drop out to the sides in a wide straddle. Your heels should be as close to your groin as possible.

3. Exhale and slowly walk your hands forward, lowering your torso towards the floor. Your forearms can rest on the floor, or you can clasp your hands behind your back.

4. Once your torso is parallel to the floor, slowly lower your head and upper body towards the mat, keeping your elbows on the floor if possible.

5. Your forehead should ideally touch the floor, creating a deep stretch in the hips, groin, and lower back. Breathe deeply and hold the pose for 5-10 breaths, focusing on relaxing into the stretch and releasing any tension in your body.

6. To release, inhale and use your core strength to slowly lift your torso back to an upright seated position.

Swan Pose (Eka Pada Rajakapotasana Variation)

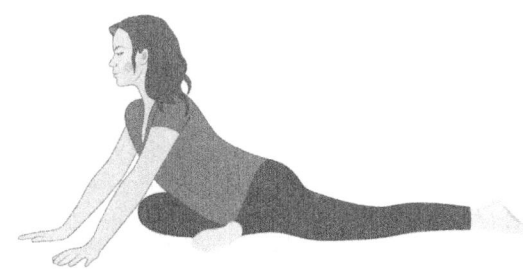

Swan Pose is an advanced backbend that requires significant flexibility and strength. It is a variation of the Pigeon Pose and should be approached with caution.

1. Begin in a low lunge position with your right leg forward and your left leg extended behind you.

2. Lower your torso towards the floor, resting your forearms on the mat and allowing your head to touch the floor if possible.

3. Exhale and lift your left leg off the floor, bending your knee and reaching back with your left hand to grab your left foot or ankle.

4. Inhale and use your core strength to lift your left leg towards the ceiling, creating a deep backbend in your spine.

5. Keep your right leg grounded and engage your quadriceps to support the pose.

6. Breathe deeply and hold the pose for 5-10 breaths, focusing on lengthening your spine and opening your chest.

7. To release, exhale and slowly lower your left leg back to the floor, then lift your torso back to the starting lunge position.

8. Repeat the pose on the other side.

Puppy Pose (Uttana Shishosana)

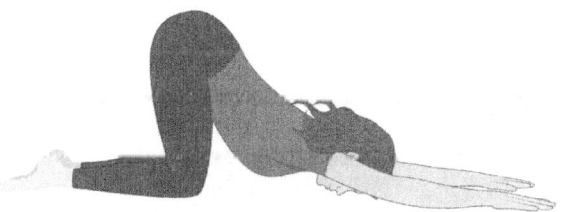

Puppy Pose is a gentle inversion that stretches the spine, shoulders, and hips while also promoting relaxation.

1. Begin on your hands and knees in a tabletop position, with your hands directly under your shoulders and your knees under your hips.

2. Walk your hands forward, allowing your chest to lower towards the floor and your hips to raise towards the ceiling.

3. As you move your torso forward, straighten your arms and create a gentle backbend in your spine.

4. Your forehead can rest on the floor, or you can keep a slight tucking of your chin to maintain the length of your neck.

5. Relax your shoulders away from your ears and allow your chest to sink towards the floor, creating a deep stretch in your upper back and shoulders.

6. Breathe deeply and hold the pose for 5-10 breaths, focusing on releasing any tension in your body and allowing gravity to deepen the stretch.

7. To release, inhale and use your core strength to lift your torso back to the starting tabletop position.

Sphinx Shoulder Opener

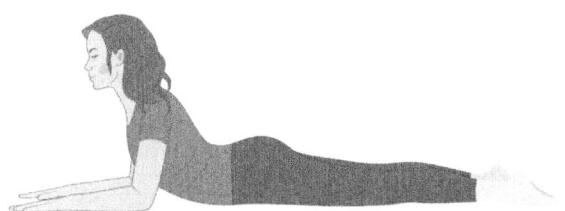

The Sphinx Shoulder Opener is a gentle backbend that stretches the shoulders, chest, and abdomen while strengthening the back muscles.

1. Lie on your stomach with your legs extended behind you, hip-width apart. Your toes can be tucked under or pointed back.

2. Bring your elbows in line with your shoulders and place your forearms on the mat, parallel to each other and forming a 90-degree angle with your upper arms.

3. Inhale and press your forearms and hands into the mat, using your back muscles to lift your chest and upper body off the floor.

4. Keep your low abdomen and hip bones anchored to the mat, creating a gentle backbend in your upper body.

5. Relax your shoulders down and away from your ears, and gently squeeze your shoulder blades together to open your chest.

6. Breathe deeply and hold the pose for 5-10 breaths, focusing on lengthening your spine and creating space between your shoulder blades.

7. To deepen the stretch, you can gently turn your head from side to side or lift your gaze towards the ceiling.

8. To release the pose, exhale and slowly lower your torso back to the mat.

Cobra Shoulder Stretch

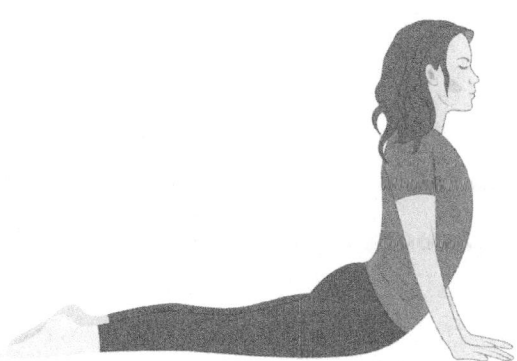

The Cobra Shoulder Stretch is a variation of the traditional Cobra Pose that targets the shoulders, upper back, and chest.

1. Begin in a prone position (lying on your stomach) with your legs extended behind you and your hands placed directly under your shoulders.

2. Inhale and press your hands into the mat, using your back muscles to lift your chest and upper body off the floor. Keep your low abdomen and hip bones anchored to the mat.

3. Straighten your arms and lift your chest higher, allowing your head to tilt back gently.

4. Squeeze your shoulder blades together, engaging your upper back muscles and creating a gentle backbend.

5. Inhale and reach your right arm forward, parallel to the floor, while simultaneously turning your torso to the right, creating a twist in your upper body.

6. Hold the twist for a few breaths, focusing on opening your right shoulder and chest.

7. Exhale and return to the center, then repeat the twist on the left side, reaching your left arm forward.

8. Continue alternating the twists for 5-10 breaths, synchronizing your movements with your breath.

9. To release, exhale and slowly lower your torso back to the mat.

Remember to move slowly and mindfully, and adjust the intensity of the poses to suit your flexibility and comfort level. Use props or modifications as needed to avoid strain or discomfort.

Balance Poses

Among the many gifts that yoga offers, developing a sense of balanced poise and grounded presence is one of the most profound. The balance poses, or asanas, challenge us to maintain physical and mental equilibrium while testing the limits of our concentration and calm.

More than just strengthening the tiny stabilizer muscles, they require us to bring all of our faculties into harmonious alignment, breath, focus, strength, and flexibility. As we still the fluctuations of the mind and body, we tap into a state of tranquil alertness and being. The balancing postures reveal areas where we grip or tense unnecessarily, and teach us to find sustainable, centered effort.

Whether balancing on two feet or one, with or without the support of our arms, the balance poses refine our proprioception—our sense of where our bodies are in space. This spatial intelligence enhances grace, agility, and mindfulness both on and off the mat. As we commit to steady surrender in the face of potential wobbles, we meet challenges with poise instead of bracing.

Tree Pose with Arms to the Sky(Vrksasana)

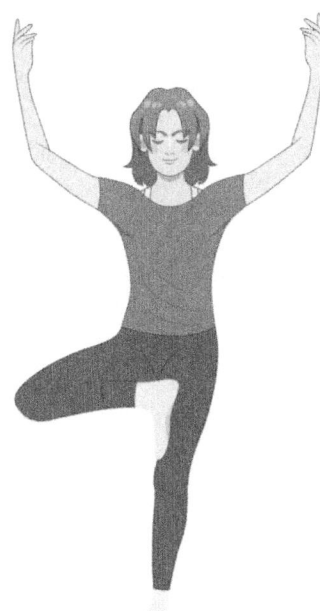

The tree pose is one of the most renowned standing balance poses in yoga. It cultivates focused steadiness while strengthening the legs, ankles, and core. In this variation, we'll be extending the arms overhead, further challenging our sense of equilibrium.

1. Stand in Mountain Pose (Tadasana), with your weight evenly distributed through your feet. Find a steady gazing point to fix your drishti (focused gaze).

2. Shift your weight onto your left foot, engaging your left thigh muscles. Bend your right knee out to the side and use your hands to place the right foot high on your left inner thigh. Avoid pressing the foot directly into the knee joint.

3. Once your right foot is secure, bring your hands together in a prayer position (Anjali Mudra) in front of your chest. This helps engage your core.

4. Inhale and sweep your arms overhead, perpendicular to the floor, with your biceps framing your ears. Open your palms to the sky, spreading your fingers wide.

5. Fix your gaze softly at a point ahead to maintain focus. Engage your standing leg, drawing energy from the earth through your foot.

6. Take 5-10 deep breaths here, staying centered over your standing leg. If you feel steady, you can alternate between looking up at your hands and keeping a forward gaze.

7. To release, exhale, and bring your hands back to prayer. Use your hands to release your foot back to the mat. Repeat on the other side.

Move slowly with your breath. If you lose your balance, just step out and reset before trying again. Tree pose strengthens focus amidst constant micro-adjustments.

Warrior III (Virabhadrasana III)

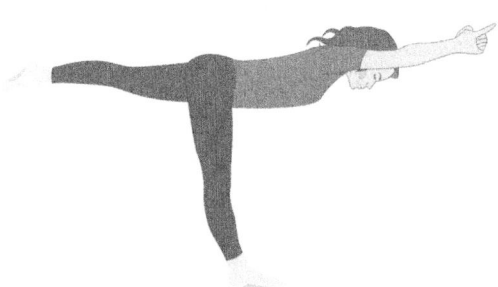

Warrior III challenges your balance, strength, and concentration in an asymmetrical arm and leg extension. This grounded, yet energizing posture helps build stamina while developing calm focus.

1. Stand at the front of your mat in Mountain Pose (Tadasana). Bring your weight onto the left foot, keeping the left leg straight with your left knee unlocked.

2. Shift your body weight forward over the left leg as you lift the right leg off the floor behind you, keeping the right leg straight and strong. Allow the torso to hinge forward from the hip joints.

3. Extend the right leg back in a straight line from the hip, while simultaneously stretching the arms forward in line with the ears. Engage the right leg and reach strongly back through the right heel.

4. Keep the front knee unlocked by micro-bending it. Lengthen the tailbone toward the back heel to maintain extension through both legs.

5. Direct your gaze slightly ahead of you to help keep the body in one line. Take 5-8 deep, steady breaths.

6. Engage your core by activating your navel toward the spine. Root down through the standing foot to find steadiness.

7. To release, bring the right foot back to the floor with control on an exhalation. Pause, then repeat on the other side.

8. Go slowly and focus on alignment over depth. Use a wall for support if needed as you build strength. Feel the union of stability and mobility as you embody the focused power of the warrior.

Kneeling Half Moon Pose (Ardha Chandrasana)

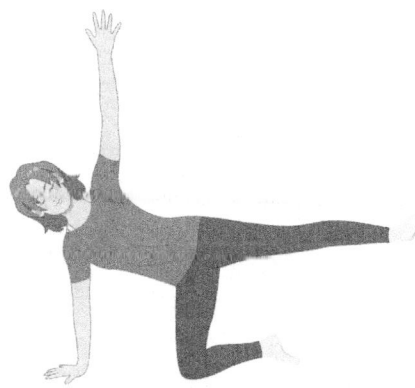

This grounded side bend asks you to find length, openness, and balance on one side of the body. Kneeling Half Moon cultivates focus, stability in the base, and freedom in the upper body.

1. Start in a low kneeling lunge position, with your right knee directly under your right hip and your left foot positioned between your right calf and thigh. Untuck your left toes.

2. Put your hands on your hips and lengthen through your torso, finding a neutral spine. Root down through your right knee.

3. Inhale and raise your left arm toward the ceiling, actively reaching your fingertips up. Keep your right hand on your right hip.

4. As you exhale, lean your upper body over to the left, reaching your left fingertips down and across your body. Let your head turn to gaze at your left thumb.

5. Press your right foot firmly into the mat to stabilize your base. Engage your core by drawing your navel toward your spine.

6. Take 5-7 deep breaths, finding length on both sides of your torso. For more of a bind, reach your right arm forward along the mat.

7. To release, inhale and return to the center. Switch sides, kneeling the left leg forward.

Find steady openness, not straining or over-efforting. Distribute your weight evenly between your kneeling knee and foot. Let your spine elongate in this balanced side bend. Use a block under your hand if needed.

Eagle Arms Close-Up

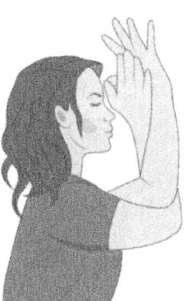

This arm variation of the balancing Eagle Pose requires concentration and upper body strength as you twist, and bend the arms. It challenges your focus and tests your patience.

1. Begin in a standing position, with your feet parallel or slightly pigeon-toed if needed for stability. Draw your shoulder blades down your back.

2. Raise your arms parallel to the floor, bending at the elbows so your forearms are perpendicular.

3. Keeping the elbows raised, cross one forearm over the other and hook the hands to create an eagle embrace. Your palms can stay open or make fists.

4. On an inhalation, draw the crossed arms closer toward your face, keeping the shoulders relaxed and elbows lifted.

5. Hold your drishti (focused gaze) steadily ahead to maintain balance. Take a few grounding breaths.

6. For an added challenge, keep hugging the arms as you raise them overhead, stacking the elbows directly over the wrists.

7. Hold for 5-8 steady breaths. Then unwind by reversing the arm cross and release.

Move slowly and mindfully to avoid pinching in the shoulders. Modify by only bringing the arms halfway or using a strap for the bind. The closeness of the arms challenges proprioception and steadiness of the mind. Stay patient yet lighthearted as you awaken new spaces.

Dancer's Pose (Natarajasana)

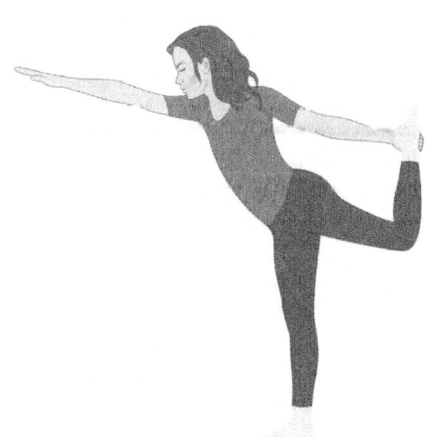

This arm variation of the balancing Eagle Pose requires concentration and upper body strength as you twist and bind the arms.

1. Begin in a standing position, with your feet parallel or slightly pigeon-toed if needed for stability. Draw your shoulder blades down your back.

2. Raise your arms parallel to the floor, bending at the elbows so your forearms are perpendicular.

3. Keeping the elbows raised, cross one forearm over the other and hook the hands to create an eagle embrace. Your palms can stay open or make fists.

4. On an inhalation, draw the crossed arms closer toward your face, keeping the shoulders relaxed and elbows lifted.

5. Hold your drishti (focused gaze) steadily ahead to maintain balance. Take a few grounding breaths.

6. For an added challenge, keep hugging the arms as you raise them overhead, stacking the elbows directly over the wrists.

7. Hold for 5-8 steady breaths. Then unwind by reversing the arm cross and release.

Move slowly and mindfully to avoid pinching in the shoulders. Modify by only bringing the arms halfway or using a strap for the bind. The closeness of the arms challenges proprioception and steadiness of the mind. Stay patient yet lighthearted as you awaken new spaces.

Standing Splits (Urdhva Prasarita Eka Padasana)

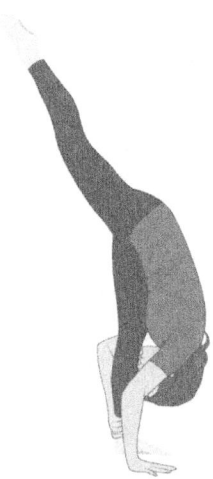

This gravity-defying balancing tests your focus, flexibility, and core control as you take one leg skyward into a standing split position.

1. Begin standing in Tadasana (Mountain Pose). Shift your weight onto your left foot, engaging your quadriceps.

2. On an inhalation, raise your right leg out in front of you, actively lifting from the hip crease. Use your hands on your right leg to help get height.

3. Keep your standing leg deeply rooted as you extend the raised leg toward the ceiling, creating one straight line of energy from your heel to your fingertips.

4. Once extended, release your hands and reach your arms alongside your ears, framing your face. Fix your drishti (focused gaze) softly ahead.

5. Engage your core by drawing your low belly inward. This will help prevent arching in your lower back.

6. Take 5-8 steady breaths, softening the weight of the head and finding length through the spine.

7. To release, bend your standing knee and bring your hands to your raised leg. Slowly release it back to the mat with control.

Don't worry about perfect split flexibility—honor where your body is today. Use a wall for assistance if needed. The real challenge is maintaining a single-point focus and core engagement.

One-Legged Mountain Pose (Eka Pada Tadasana)

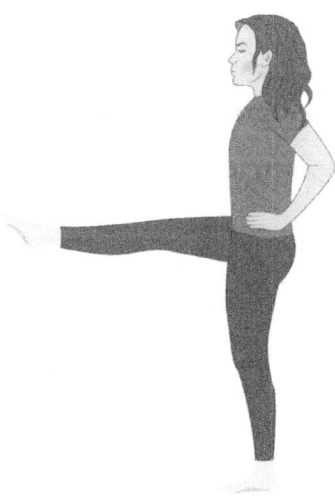

1. In Mountain Pose (Tadasana) with your feet together and weight evenly distributed, find a focused drishti point ahead.

2. Carry your weight onto your left foot, engaging your quadriceps. Keep your left knee soft, not locked.

3. On an inhalation, lift your right foot off the floor. Bring the sole of the right foot to the left ankle, shin, or inner thigh—avoid the knee joint. Let your hands rest on your hips.

4. Root down with conviction through your standing foot. Imagine energetic roots extending from your foot into the earth.

5. Engage your core by drawing your navel inward toward your spine. Keep your chest lifted.

6. Take 5-10 steady breaths here, softening the shoulders and jaw. You can raise your arms overhead for an added challenge.

7. To release, mindfully place your raised foot back on the mat with control.

Focus on the quality of your foundation rather than the height of the leg. A steady, even breath will help you find your center of gravity. Play with micro-adjustments and core engagement to cultivate unwavering concentration.

Warrior III with Arms Forward

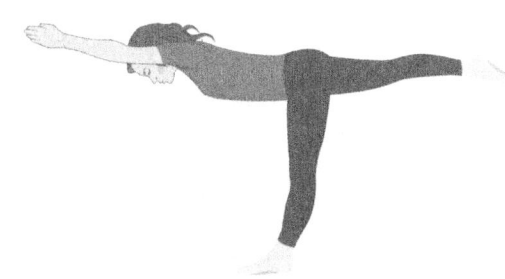

This advanced variation of the Warrior III pose challenges your balance, core strength, and focus as you extend your arms forward instead of alongside your body. Prepare to feel energized yet grounded.

1. Start in Warrior I (Virabhadrasana I) with your left foot forward, and legs in a wide stance. Root down through your feet.

2. Exhale and shift your weight forward over your front foot as you raise your back heel off the mat, coming into Warrior III alignment.

3. Extend your arms forward in line with your ears, actively reaching the fingertips away from the shoulders. Avoid hunching the shoulders.

4. Lengthen your tailbone toward the wall behind you and engage your quadriceps to straighten your front leg.

5. Lift your gaze softly forward to help keep your spine in one long line. Take a few deep breaths

6. Engage your core strongly by drawing your navel toward your spine. Imagine a string pulling you forward from the center of your chest.

7. Breathe smoothly for 5-8 rounds, finding steadiness. To release, mindfully place your back foot down with control.

8. Go slowly as you build the strength for this arm variation. Focus on extension from fingertips to heels rather than depth. Use a wall or door frame to assist with balance if needed. Feel simultaneously energized and rooted.

Tree Pose with Side Bend

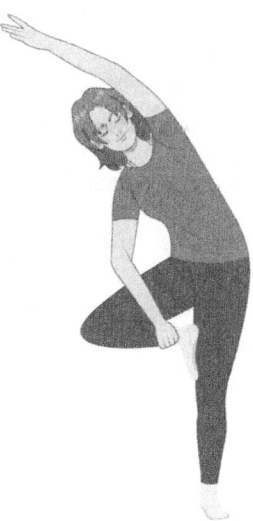

This balancing variation of Tree Pose adds a lateral side bend, further challenging your focus and stability. It opens the sides of the body while developing core control.

1. Start with Tree Pose (Vrksasana) with your right foot rooted against your left inner thigh and hands in prayer position at your chest.

2. Once stable, inhale and raise your right arm overhead, bicep by ear, reaching through your right fingertips.

3. As you exhale, laterally bend your upper body over to the left, reaching your left fingertips toward the floor. Avoid hunching your shoulders.

4. Keep your core engaged by drawing your navel inward. Allow your head to turn so your gaze follows your left fingertips.

5. Take 5-7 deep breaths here, focusing on lengthening the entire right side body from heel to fingertips.

6. Avoid gripping. Let your left hip release toward the left to facilitate the side bend.

7. To release, inhale back to the center Tree, then lower your right foot.

Move slowly with your breath. Modify by only lifting your bottom arm or using a wall for support. Concentrate on maintaining internal body alignment as you bend sideways. Go easy into any intensity—the real challenge is stillness within the motion.

Standing Figure Four Stretch

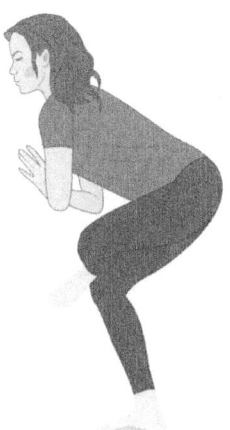

This balancing stretch opens the hips while testing your ability to stay centered and focused. It provides an intense outer hip release in an asymmetrical standing posture.

1. Begin standing in Mountain Pose (Tadasana). Cross your right ankle over your left thigh, creating a figure-4 shape with your legs. Allow your right knee to open out to the side.

2. Flex through your left foot to root down as you bend your standing knee. Only bend as far as you can while keeping your heel grounded.

3. On an inhale, raise your arms overhead, biceps framing your ears. Fix your gaze ahead to find a drishti point.

4. Engage your core by drawing your navel inward. This will prevent you from collapsing into your lower back.

5. Take 5-8 deep breaths, concentrating on stacking your left hip over your left ankle. You can hold onto a wall if needed.

6. Go easy into any intensity by only bending your standing knee as far as is comfortable.

7. To release, place your hands on your hips and slowly unwind to stand.

Move mindfully, as this shape can be intense for the outer hips and knees. Listen to your body and back off if you feel any pinching discomfort. Focus on rooting down through your standing leg to create stable freedom in your hip.

Chapter Six

28 Days to Weight Loss and A Stress-Free Life

Good things like good friendships, relationships, and good health don't just fall on our laps; we have to work towards them. The quest for physical well-being is often filled with twists, turns, and obstacles that can test our resolve. That's why committing to a holistic program like this 28-day Somatic Yoga practice is so powerful.

It's not just about shedding pounds or building strength, although those are certainly wonderful side effects. This program is about cultivating a deep, nurturing relationship with yourself–a relationship built on self-compassion, mindfulness, and a willingness to show up fully for your own growth and healing.

Over the next 28 days, you'll be invited to move beyond the harsh, critical voices that so often dominate our inner dialogues. Instead, you'll learn to embrace a kinder, more forgiving perspective–one that celebrates your courage for stepping onto this path and honors the beautiful, messy complexity of the human experience.

Each day's practice will move you closer to a deeper state of relaxation, where you can begin to untangle the knots of stress, anxiety, and self-doubt that may have held you back in the past. With patience, persistence, and a generous dose of self-love, you'll discover the profound wisdom that lives within your body, mind, and spirit.

Week 1

Day 1: Establishing Presence

- Breath Work: 3-Part Breath (5 mins)

- Gentle Warm-Up: Cat/Cow, Knee Hugs (5 mins)
- Child's Pose (3 mins)
- Easy Seat - Body Scan Meditation (10 mins)
- Savasana (5 mins)

Day 2: Rest

Day 3: Core Awakening

- Breath Work (3 mins)
- Warm-Up: Cat/Cow, Knee Hugs, Arm Circles (5 mins)
- Boat Pose (5 breaths)
- Locust Variations (5 on each side)
- Upward Plank (5 breaths)
- Savasana (7 mins)

Day 4: Rest

Day 5: Finding Your Foundation

- Breath Work (3 mins)
- Sun Salutation A (3 rounds)
- Mountain Pose (5 breaths)
- Forward Fold (8 breaths)
- Half Sun Salutation (3 on each side)
- Savasana (5 mins)

Day 6: Rest

Day 7: Softening & Surrendering

- Breath Work (5 mins)

- Warm-Up: Cat/Cow, Knee Hugs (3 mins)
- Wide-Legged Forward Fold (8 breaths)
- Seated Forward Fold (10 breaths)
- Supine Twist (5 on each side)
- Savasana (10 mins)

Week 2: Building Strength and Stability

Day 8: Awakening the Warrior

- Breath Work (5 mins)
- Sun Salutations A & B (5 rounds)
- Warrior I (8 breaths per side)
- Warrior II (8 breaths per side)
- Reverse Warrior (5 breaths per side)
- Savasana (7 mins)

Day 9: Rest

Day 10: Fortifying the Core

- Breath Work (3 mins)
- Warm Up: Cat/Cow, Knee Hugs (5 mins)
- Boat Pose (10 breaths)
- Plank Pose (8 breaths)
- Side Plank (5 breaths per side)
- Savasana (5 mins)

Day 11: Rest

Day 12: Balance and Stability

- Breath Work (3 mins)
- Sun Salutation C (3 rounds)
- Tree Pose (8 breaths per side)
- Eagle Pose (5 breaths per side)
- Dancer's Pose (8 breaths per side)
- Savasana (7 mins)

Day 13: Rest

Day 14: Grounding and Rooting

- Breath Work (5 mins)
- Warm Up: Hip Circles (3 mins)
- Malasana/Yogi Squat (10 breaths)
- Chair Pose (8 breaths)
- Standing Forward Fold (10 breaths)
- Savasana (8 mins)

Week 3: Releasing Tension and Stress

Day 15: Unwinding the Spine

- Breath Work (5 mins)
- Cat/Cow (5 rounds)
- Seated Spinal Twists (5 on each side)
- Seated Forward Fold (10 breaths)
- Child's Pose (5 breaths)

- Savasana (7 mins)

Day 16: Rest

Day 17: Opening the Hips

- Breath Work (3 mins)
- Low Lunge Variations (5 breaths on each side)
- Pigeon Pose (8 breaths on each side)
- Reclining Bound Angle Pose (10 breaths)
- Savasana (8 mins)

Day 18: Rest

Day 19: Softening the Shoulders

- Breath Work (5 mins)
- Arm Circles & Shoulder Rolls (3 mins)
- Extended Puppy Pose (8 breaths)
- Reverse Prayer Pose (5 breaths)
- Savasana (7 mins)

Day 20: Rest

Day 21: Deep Relaxation

- Breath Work (3 mins)
- Gentle Seated Twists (5 on each side)
- Legs Up The Wall Pose (10 mins)
- Savasana (12 mins)

Week 4: Integration and Transformation

Day 22: Balancing Mind & Body

- Breath Work: Alternate Nostril (5 mins)
- Sun Salutations A & B (3 rounds)
- Tree Pose (5 breaths per side)
- Warrior III (8 breaths per side)
- Balance Sequence: Eagle, Dancer's Pose (5 breaths each)
- Savasana (7 mins)

Day 23: Rest

Day 24: Mindful Movement

- Body Scan Meditation (10 mins)
- Gentle Yoga Flow focused on breath awareness (20 mins)
- Savasana (10 mins)

Day 25: Rest

Day 26: Uniting Strength & Surrender

- Breath Work: Kapalabhati (3 mins)
- Strength Poses: Plank, Side Plank, Upward Plank (5 breaths each)
- Forward Folds: Wide Stance, Seated (8 breaths each)
- Savasana (10 mins)

Day 27: Rest

Day 28: Self-Renewal

- Breath work (7 mins)

- Mindful Meditation (15 mins)
- Gentle Stretches & Savasana (15 mins)
- Reflection/Closing Ceremony

Chapter Seven

Tracking Your Somatic Journey

There's something quite incredible about intention. About choosing to show up and to do your best even when it's so hard. About declaring and defining that this is what I want, and I am going to work towards it with everything in me until I take my last breath.

Those first few steps that we take when we start something are always the hardest, every part of us is tempted to cling to the familiar, to stay rooted in what's comfortable and known, even if it's not serving us well; but there's always something inside that knows that there's more, that we're worthy of more, that we're capable of more if we're willing to lean into the discomfort.

And so we start. We start by committing ourselves, a promise to tend to our becoming. We clear space on our calendars and in our minds for what's ahead. We gather the tools and allies that will support us along the way–the yoga mat, the journal, and the community cheering us on.

There will be amazing days where everything clicks, and brutal days where we question if we have what it takes, but that's precisely why tracking your somatic journey is so powerful, it gives you a tangible record of your growth, your breakthroughs, your "aha" moments. When you take the time to notice and document how you're feeling physically, mentally, and emotionally–you create an invaluable map that can guide you back to your truth when the way forward feels uncertain. Those journal entries become monuments to your resilience, reminding you of the progress you've made and the wisdom you've unearthed, one courageous step at a time.

Embrace this process of tracking, not as a chore or obligation, but as a celebration of your wholehearted commitment to this journey. Let it be an anchor to your intentions, a mirror reflecting your immense strength and beauty to you, a compass ever-pointing you towards your healthiest self.

Setting Intentions

At the heart of anything is the intention of that blazing spark of desire that compels us forward even when the path feels arduous. Intentions are the beacons that light our way, reminding us of our "why" and refocusing our energy on what truly matters. They are, however, not the same as goals or resolutions. Those are specific milestones and targets we set for ourselves. Intentions run deeper—they are the felt experiences, qualities, and ways of being that we wish to embody and inhabit more fully in our lives.

Maybe you intend to approach yourself and your practice with more compassion instead of harsh self-criticism. Maybe it's to cultivate a deeper sense of presence amidst the frenzy of modern life. Or perhaps you intend to experience more freedom and lightness in your body, unburdened by limiting beliefs.

When we set intentions from this soulful, open-hearted space, they become powerful catalysts for that inner shift. Here are some tips for setting intentions that will nourish your journey.

- Get clear on your core desired feelings. How do you want to feel as you move through your exercises? Anchored, vibrant, peaceful, healthy, and empowered in your body?

- Keep intentions positive. "Let go of anxiety" can become "open myself to the comfort of being in my body."

- Use present tense. "I am patient with my growth." This plants the seed in your subconscious mind.

- Be specific but not rigid. "to welcome joy when joy comes" rather than "be joyful all the time."

- Most importantly, set intentions without attachment to the outcome. They are invitations for change, not demands.

So take a few grounding breaths, place a hand over your heart, and ask yourself—what intentions are yearning to blossom in my life right now? The answers may surprise you.

Journaling Your Experience

Your journal holds the beautiful complexity of this whole without judgment or agenda. It's a confidant, a mirror, a time capsule of what's in your soul and heart.

When you take the time to reflect through writing, you forge a deeper connection with yourself. The act of putting pen to paper sparks an alchemical unraveling within. Thoughts become clearer, emotions flow more freely, and your inner voice, so often muted by external noise, begins to bloom in vibrancy.

As you re-read past entries, you'll marvel at how far you've come. You'll be a witness to the dedicated person that you are. In this sense, your journal becomes a tangible map, tracing the terrain of your awakening consciousness.

To fully benefit from this explorative process, try embracing a few journal tips.

- Notice physical sensations. After practice, take a few minutes to tune into your body and jot down any areas of ease, tension, openness, or restriction you noticed.

- Explore emotional landscapes. Somatic work inevitably stirs up feelings. Note any emotions that surfaced and how they manifested physically.

- Track progress over time. Periodically re-read previous entries to see how your experience of poses, breathing exercises, or meditations has shifted.

- Include somatic inquiries. Use your journal to note questions for further contemplation like "What am I holding in my belly/shoulders/jaw?" or "Where am I resisting softening?"

- Detail embodied insights. Somatic work reveals wisdom. Capture any "aha" moments about your patterns, habits, or core beliefs.

- Reflect on challenges. If you struggle through a practice, explore what came up for you with curiosity and self-compassion.

- Let it be a playground. Don't just record—interact with your pages through sketches, mind maps, or creative writing exercises.

- Most of all, let your journal be a sacred, non-judgmental container for your somatic exploration. This is a place of radical honesty and self-discovery.

Take your practice to deeper levels by downloading the free **Tracking Journal**. This beautifully designed digital journal allows you to record your experiences, insights, emotions, and progress over time. With dedicated sections for noting physical sensations, emotional landscapes, inquiries, and "aha" moments, it becomes an invaluable companion on your somatic journey.

Tracking Physical Changes

You are likely going to notice shifts happening not just in your mind and heart, but in your physical beingness as well. You might start to stand a little taller, movements feeling more easeful as you release long-held tensions. Or maybe you'll find joy in newfound strength and stability, no longer held back by habits of collapsing or gripping. Some of you may even experience a gradual shedding of excess weight as you attune more deeply to your body's innate wisdom.

Regardless of the specific changes, taking the time to consciously track your physical progress can be incredibly empowering and motivating. It provides unequivocal evidence of your commitment to actively reshaping your life in alignment with your highest intentions.

- Take monthly photos from the same angles to visually document changes over time.

- Note shifts in clothing fit, muscle tone, flexibility, and stamina.
- Keep a log of goals like holding a pose longer or achieving a new strength milestone.
- Enlist friends or family to share observations about your posture/presence.
- Most importantly, focus on how you feel rather than numeric tracking metrics. The scale's story is incredibly limited.
- Notice the quality of your breath—does it feel more fluid and spacious?
- Tune into your energy levels throughout the day as you become more embodied.

This isn't about criticism or judgment, but radical self-attunement. You're gathering data that reflects the profound work happening at every level of your being. So celebrate each small and large victory as a renewal of your vows to fully inhabit this one precious life. Let the toning muscle, the uplifted gaze, and the easier way of moving through the world be reminders that you are remaking yourself with every intentional breath and step. What an awesome responsibility and privilege.

Reflecting on Emotional Shifts

Emotional shifts are inevitable, after all, buried beneath the layers of physical tension and holding patterns, emotional blockages and wounds are crying out for acknowledgment, compassion, and release.

This somatic work creates an opportunity to forge an entirely new relationship with your emotional landscape. Instead of suppressing, avoiding, or forcefully "muscling through" difficult feelings, you learn to greet them with exquisite tenderness. To let them flow, alchemize, and guide you towards deeper self-acceptance and freedom; you create referenceable treasures that map your resilience over time because make no mistake, recognizing, metabolizing, and integrating challenging emotions is some of the best work you'll ever do.

- Note the emotions that arise and any accompanying physical sensations like tightness or temperature changes.
- Explore the habitual thought patterns, core beliefs, or memories that may be

fueling those emotions.

- Don't judge or analyze - simply have compassionate awareness of what you're experiencing.

- Let your journal be an outlet to freely emote through prose, poetry or even sketching your "feeling" iconography.

- Most importantly, celebrate any expansions in your ability to feel, express, and process your emotions fully. That is true freedom.

As you become more at home in your emotional depths, you'll start viewing feelings, even the difficult ones, as navigational aids rather than inconveniences. They'll reveal where you're getting hooked and constricted, shining light on paths toward greater openness, authenticity, and liberation.

So let your journal pages become realms of intimate self-discovery. Places where you can peel back the layers, visit the tender spaces within, and come back ever more sovereign in your emotional fluidity and radiance.

Conclusion

I live for the days when I wake up thinking, "Oh wow, I didn't know that being alive could ever feel this good." Those precious moments when my body feels light, my mind is clear, and my spirit is soaring. Over the years, I've learned to embrace all the layers of my being—the physical, mental, and emotional. This holistic approach has been key in teaching me to move with intention, breathe with presence, and approach each posture as a sacred dance between mind, body, and soul.

I don't want you to simply read these words; I want you to feel them resonating within the very depths of your heart because that's what somatic yoga is all about – feeling deeply, connecting profoundly, and awakening to the vast expanses of your inner landscape.

We've explored the art of cultivating awareness, moving beyond the physical realm, and tapping into the whisperings of our souls. We've learned to shed the layers of tension, stress, and self-doubt that so often weigh us down, and instead, embrace the freedom of living in harmony with our authentic selves.

And while the journey hasn't always been easy—after all, true growth rarely occurs without some discomfort—I hope to rest in the knowledge that you are not alone. We are all works in progress, forever evolving, forever learning to love and accept ourselves more fully with each breath, each movement, and each conscious choice to show up for our lives.

As you carry these teachings forward, remember that somatic yoga is simply but a way of being—a lens through which to view the world with compassion, curiosity, and an unwavering belief in your inherent worth. I hope that this book will be a constant reminder to honor your body's wisdom, to listen to the whispers of your soul, and to move through this world with grace, courage, and an unshakable commitment to living your most vibrant, authentic life because when we learn to embody our truest selves, that's when the magic happens—that's when we wake up thinking, "Oh wow, I didn't know that being alive could ever feel this good."

If you felt that this book truly resonated with you, I'd be so grateful if you left a review, who knows, it might just be the very reason why this book ends up in the hands of another hopeful reader like you.

Exercise Index

Mountain Pose 35

Forward Fold 36

Warrior I 37

Warrior II 38

Extended Side Angle Pose 39

Tree Pose 40

Chair Pose 41

Crescent Lunge Pose 42

Half Moon Pose 43

Eagle Pose 44

Seated Forward Fold (Paschimottanasana) 46

Butterfly Pose (Baddha Konasana) 47

Seated Twist (Ardha Matsyendrasana) 48

Boat Pose (va-asana) 49

Wide-Legged Forward Fold (Upavistha Nonasana) 50

Seated Wide-Legged Straddle (Upavistha Nonasana) 51

Half Lord of the Fishes Pose (Ardha Matsyendrasana) 52

Cow Face Pose (Gomukhasana) 53

Seated Forward Bend with Legs Crossed 54

Seated Spinal Twist (Marichyasana) 55

Reclining Bound Angle Pose 56

Supine Spinal Twist (Supta Matsyendrasana) 58

Happy Babe Pose (Ananda Balasana) 59

SuGine Figure Four Stretch (Supine Pigeon Pose) 61

Legs Up the Wall Pose (Viparita Karani) 62

Reclining Hero Pose (Supta Virasana) 63

Reclining Bound Angle Twist 64

Supine Butterfly Stretch 65

Reclining Hamstring Stretch 66

Sphinx Pose (Salamba Bhujangasana) 68

Cobra Pose (Bhujangasana) 69

Locust Pose (Salajhasana) 70

Bow Pose (Ohanurasana) 71

Baby Cobra Pose (Ardha Bhujangasana) 72

Crocodile Pose (Makarasana) 73

Swan Pose 74

Puppy Pose (Uttana Shishosana) 75

Sphinx Shoulder Opener 76

Cobra Shoulder Stretch 77

Tree Pose with Arms to the Sky 78

Warrior III (Virabhadrasana III) 80

Kneeling Half Moon Pose (Ardha Chandrasana) 81

Eagle Arms Close-Up 82

Dancer's Pose (Natarajasana) 83

Standing Splits 84

One-Legged Mountain Pose 85

Warrior III with Arms Forward 86

Tree Pose with Side Bend 87

Standing Figure Four Stretch 88

Printed in Great Britain
by Amazon